THE
Vitamin D
CURE

Revised Edition

James Dowd, M.D.

Diane Stafford

WILEY

John Wiley & Sons, Inc.

To my patients, my family, and my dogs
—James Dowd, M.D.

To Greg—thanks for your wonderful love and support.
—Diane Stafford

Contents

Acknowledgments

Twice a year I write a one-page newsletter to physicians who refer patients to me, and one fall I decided to include information on vitamin D deficiency. At the time, I had only a basic knowledge of vitamin D. I'd seen one woman who had obesity, arthritis, mood disturbance, and chronic pain. She was severely vitamin D–deficient, but all of her symptoms improved when I put her on vitamin D supplements.

I began studying vitamin D for the newsletter, and that was when a whole new perspective on medicine opened up for me. It was as if I had discovered an ocean that connected all my islands of knowledge, and I'd just received a free pass on a ship that could navigate these seas.

We all struggle to live our lives with purpose, but it's really something special when purpose finds us and carries us on an unexpected journey. In this case, the ships that have carried me on this journey have crews, and I cannot thank them enough for the excitement they have returned to my practice of medicine.

Michael Holick's research introduced me to this incredible hormone. As I pored over the scientific literature, I began to meet the researchers who have spent their entire careers studying vitamin D, many of whom passed on their passion to a younger generation of scientists—people such as Robert Heaney, Anthony Norman, Bruce Hollis, Reinhold Vieth, Cedric Garland, Gary Schwartz, Barbara Boucher, Norman Bell, Armin Zittermann, Bess Dawson-Hughes, Susan Harris,

Ann Looker, Heike Bischoff-Ferrari, Margherita Cantorna, Rolf Jorde, William Grant, John Cannell, and Captain Hector DeLuca. So many have learned so much from Hector DeLuca. And there are many more.

As I began to apply what I learned about vitamin D, I found that while many patients felt better after starting supplements, many did *not*, which led me to explore calcium balance and the factors that influenced this mineral beyond vitamin D. It seems I had stepped off one ship and onto another, and the journey morphed into a completely new understanding of how diet regulates body chemistry, affecting much more than our weight. The new crew included scientists and clinicians such as S. Boyd Eaton, Loren Cordain, Anthony Sebastian, Lynda Frassetto, Friedrich Manz, Thomas Remer, Jürgen Vormann, Charles Pak, Khashayar Sakhaee, Artemis Simopoulos, Jane Kerstetter, David Barker, Peter Gluckman, and most recently, Jeffrey Gordon. These scientists and clinicians have changed my life.

This book was my chance to share my excitement and what I have brought to my practice with a larger audience. It fulfills the main reason why I pursued a career in medicine: to help people. For this opportunity, I thank my agent, Faith Hamlin, with Sanford J. Greenburger & Associates, and my coauthor, Diane Stafford, who transformed my often dry scientific ramblings into readable prose. Finally, I would like to thank Tom Miller, our editor at John Wiley & Sons. Tom has embraced our message and has helped to craft a book that we're all excited about.

—James Dowd, M.D.

In the yearlong journey that produced this book, I worked closely with my coauthor, James Dowd, M.D., whose experiences and knowledge made this book exceptional. I have great appreciation for his Vitamin D Cure, which has made a tremendous difference in many people's lives, including mine!

Enormous gratitude goes to Faith Hamlin, our top-notch literary agent who made this book possible; Tom Miller, our editor at John Wiley & Sons, who brought his excellent insights and publishing savvy to this book; my parents, Clinton and Belle Shirley, who encouraged my way with words lifelong; my family and friends, who kept me balanced to the degree that a writer can be balanced. Love and thanks to my family, near and far, including Jenny, Ben, London, Allen, Camilla, Richard, Gina, Christina, Austin, Xanthe, Britt, Renee, Lindsay, Josh, Ella, Curt, Cameron—and my dear husband Greg, Molly, Dylan, Cita, Greg, Laura, Patrick, Katrina, Mark, Matthew, and Melinda—and all of their beautiful children, who always make me smile.

—Diane Stafford

Authors' Note

This book contains the authors' opinions and ideas based on research. It is intended to provide helpful and informative information on the subject matter covered herein. This book is sold with the understanding that the authors and the publisher are not engaged in rendering professional medical, health, or other personal professional services via this book. If the reader wants or needs personal advice, counsel, or guidance, he or she should seek an in-person consultation with a competent medical professional who has the opportunity to assess that individual's exact health history and situation. Furthermore, the reader should consult his or her medical professional before adopting any of the suggestions in the book or drawing inferences from information included herein. This is a supplement—not a replacement—for medical advice from a reader's personal health-care provider. Check with your doctor before following any recommendations in this book or before self-treating any condition that may require medical diagnosis or attention.

The authors and the publisher specifically disclaim any responsibility for any liability, loss, or risk, whether personal or otherwise, that someone may incur as a consequence, directly or indirectly, of the use and application of any of the contents of this book. In no way does reading this book replace the need for an evaluation by a physician. Also, responsibility for any adverse effects that result from the use of information in this book rests solely with the reader.

Preface to the Revised Edition

The original edition of *The Vitamin D Cure* featured some forecasts about the role that vitamin D would play in certain diseases, and these were based on the research available at the time. In the last five years, the volume of research on vitamin D has grown exponentially, and new evidence has further solidified the predictions in the original edition. This is especially true of the role vitamin D appears to play in heart and vascular disease, diabetes, infection, inflammation, mood, and memory.

Now let's take a look at what's new.

An increased risk of death from cardiovascular disease and death from all causes was linked to vitamin D deficiency when researchers analyzed information from some of the large population databases managed by Harvard University (Framingham Offspring Cohort, Health Professionals Follow-Up Study) and National Health and Nutrition Examination Survey data from the CDC. Similar studies in Germany and Norway confirmed these findings.

The role of vitamin D as an anti-inflammatory has taken center stage in age-related diseases such as cardiovascular disease, adult onset diabetes, depression, and dementia. We were aware of its importance in autoimmune diseases, but we now believe that chronic low-grade inflammation is at the heart of many adult degenerative diseases. Fueling the inflammation is our nation's pandemic of vitamin D deficiency, poor nutrition with acid base imbalance, and inactivity. But this book does offer solid solutions.

New to the revised edition are fifteen more recipes and a two-week menu. Chef Kelly, who supplies recipes for *The Vitamin D Cure Blog*, provided these recipes for the book. She has an undergraduate degree in hospitality services administration and an associate degree in culinary arts. All of her recipes have common ingredients, are easy to prepare, and follow the guidelines in *The Vitamin D Cure*. See Kelly's website at www.tastesmilerepeat.com.

Readers will also find 135 new references in this edition. Old and new references are on www.thevitamindcure.com. These are organized by chapter and linked to the National Library of Medicine. Most references have links to free full-text articles online.

Note from James Dowd, M.D.

The research and writing of this book have propelled my practice in a new direction. I have begun integrating nutrition and other lifestyle recommendations into my management of arthritis, bone, and autoimmune diseases in children and adults. My patients have welcomed this new approach, and the responses have been remarkable. The American Board of Integrative Holistic Medicine (www.abihm.org) certified me in 2010. It is my sincere hope that this new edition of *The Vitamin D Cure* will inspire you to embark on a healthy new lifestyle.

Introduction

A fifty-year-old woman named Barbara came to see me at the Arthritis Institute of Michigan. She complained of obesity and leg pain, and she had high blood pressure. When she answered questions on her symptoms, daily activities, and eating and exercise habits, I had enough information to tell me what was wrong: Barbara was one of the millions of people deficient in vitamin D—a problem that's easy to correct with sun, supplements, and diet adjustments.

I prescribed the Vitamin D Cure, Barbara started the program, and in six weeks she could hardly believe how much better she felt. No longer suffering from leg pain, she was losing weight, and her blood pressure had greatly improved. Best of all, she had pulled off all of these upgrades simply by making a few easy-to-implement changes. This sounds almost magical, but we're talking good commonsense medicine that has eluded many physicians for decades.

Now we've wrapped up the answers in this book. The answer to better health for your entire lifetime is in your hands. We hope you'll let it make a major difference in how joyfully you live.

This is a book that will fill you with optimism because you'll discover—for the first time ever—exactly how to get in charge of your health to a degree you may have never thought possible. As strangely simple as it may seem, you truly can harness the "sunshine vitamin" D and enjoy amazing and far-reaching positive effects on your health!

Many Americans today have numerous and expensive health problems, and so do our family members. This is an odd situation for the world's most affluent nation with one of the most sophisticated health-care systems. But that's where we are—and that's what we have to deal with.

When I tell you that a tiny vitamin supplement, a little sun, and some dietary fixes can alter your health dramatically, I'll bet you'll shake your head with skepticism. But stay with me for a few minutes while I present some important revelations that have convinced thousands of skeptical researchers and physicians worldwide.

Doing just a few lifestyle things differently can ward off dreaded diseases and have a dramatic effect on your health. All you have to do is give the Vitamin D Cure a chance, and the payoff will be yours—good health, a better future, and more quality time with your friends and family.

An unbalanced diet, vitamin D deficiency, and the medical problems they cause affect *more than two-thirds of the U.S. population* (about 200 million people). The chances are good that you or someone in your family—maybe even your child—figures into those scary statistics.

Today, vitamin D deficiency and dietary imbalances are pandemic. At the Arthritis Institute of Michigan, where I treat patients, 90 percent of patients who see a rheumatologist for treatment are deficient in vitamin D. Current statistics from the Centers for Disease Control and Prevention tell us that more than half of the general population is vitamin D–deficient, regardless of age. And about 70 percent of elderly Americans and 90 percent of Americans of color are vitamin D–deficient. Add to the mix those people who are overweight or obese because of dietary imbalance or inactivity, and the totals are staggering.

How Did We Go So Wrong?

For many people, health troubles started when they immigrated to North America from sunnier climates in other parts of the world. A hundred years ago, we saw a flood of immigrants from Europe and China. In the past fifty years, many immigrants have come from Mexico, India, Southeast Asia, and the Middle East, all far sunnier climates than most of the United States.

For post–World War II Americans, problems started with their movement into darker industrial cities in the Midwest and the Northeast to look for jobs. Since the 1980s, the digital revolution has moved most of us from the factory floor and physical labor to the desk, where we sit facing a computer. The problems continued as our urban transformation changed our diet. As immigrants and other Americans left their farms and began living and working in cities, their diets began to change.

Then the mechanization of the food industry compounded these dietary changes: canned and frozen produce replaced fresh fruits and vegetables. Free-range cattle gave way to feedlots. Fresh, lean meat was replaced by processed and canned meats. Foods such as canned ham—high in salt, saturated fat, and sugar—became popular, and the population explosion increased the demand for these inexpensive, well-preserved, tasty, and convenient foods.

The result of these altered lifestyles was an urbanization picture of decreased vitamin D production and increased consumption of wrong foods. These changes helped to diminish the health of many North Americans today. These are people who fill my office and the offices of doctors nationwide year round. North Americans feel too bad to enjoy all the abundance and opportunities available to us—but most have no idea what to do about the predicament.

Uncovering the Vitamin D Cure has revolutionized the way I approach treating patients. Most of my patients came to me with muscle and joint pain, back pain, sleep disturbances, severe fatigue, muscle cramps, and headaches. And many were also obese and had high blood pressure, diabetes, osteoarthritis, osteoporosis, autoimmune diseases, and/or dental problems. Most people, including physicians, would routinely attribute these symptoms and diseases to aging or genetics. They would say that time and genes were just running their course. I would routinely dispense a diagnosis and then send patients down the symptom-curbing path of anti-inflammatory drugs, pain medications, antidepressants, and sleep aids. Unfortunately, I saw that my own interventions often did little to stabilize or alleviate my patients' problems, so I searched for clues that would help me better understand this symptom/disease bundle.

That was when serendipity brought me into the loop: I began to experience some of the very same symptoms that plagued my patients. My joints started to swell and hurt in the springtime, and this soon became an annoying year-round problem that made it hard to clench my fist or shake hands. I developed muscle cramps in my legs, sleep disturbances, and fatigue. I gained weight. Just like my patients, I wondered why my body was starting to turn on me. I was relatively young. What was happening?

Now that I was the patient, I began to field theories for my health troubles. First, I suspected that my four decades of life were simply taking their toll or that my gene pool was kicking in. But I had no family history of arthritis or the other symptoms I was having. I wondered if some environmental factor was causing my health to go bad.

Then, suddenly, the pieces of the puzzle came together. I realized that my springtime joint stiffness had begun three years after I moved from Texas to Michigan. I had gone from a sunny climate to a darker one, and my symptoms had progressed every year after that. At the same time, my diet had changed. I was eating foods richer in salt, pasta, bread, cereal, and cheese. I exercised less and moved infrequently—I'd hired a gardener so I wouldn't have to spend my day off doing yard work. Lifestyle changes—could they be the culprits?

The truth finally kicked in: I was a vitamin D–deficient American whose diet was a mess. I began to improve my eating habits, and I started taking vitamin D supplements. Miraculously, my symptoms disappeared in just a few months. Then I added a simple daily exercise regimen, which almost totally eliminated the back and neck pain I'd been having. I felt ten years younger.

This book carries the wonderful promise that you can do yourself the same favor. In a short time, using the Vitamin D Cure, you can make yourself well!

Check the list of symptoms and diseases in chapter 1. If you see your own nagging health bothers on those lists, get started with your own personal fixer-upper. Assess your levels of vitamin D, good nutrition, and exercise; make a few changes; and you can feel better in ninety days or less.

Follow the five-step program provided in *The Vitamin D Cure* and you can eliminate many major health issues from your list of problems. Making these positive lifestyle changes won't necessarily save your marriage or make your neighbors more neighborly or ensure that your kids never get into trouble, but this new way of living *will* make you feel worlds better, look younger, lose weight, and ward off disease.

Now let's explore the promise.

The Wonders of Vitamin D

If you're *sick and tired* of feeling sick and tired, you've picked up the right book. Vitamin D deficiency is rampant in the United States today. It's mind-boggling how many health problems have a D deficiency element.

The very important message this book conveys is that by correcting your vitamin D deficiency and fixing the acid-base imbalance in your diet, you can get a new lease on good health once and for all!

In part one we look at who needs vitamin D (hint: *everyone*), what vitamin D is, where it comes from, the connection between D and your diet, and how the Vitamin D Cure works.

1

Most of Us Need
Way More Vitamin D

Sharon came to see me because she was tired of feeling bad. She had diabetes and suffered from chronic pain and fatigue. Wintertime was especially hard because her depression was impossible to shake.

No surprises for me, of course, because I see patients like Sharon every day in my clinic. That commonality was exactly what led me to the discovery that certain symptoms and diseases have clear-cut links to vitamin D deficiency, dietary imbalance, and inactivity.

Like many of my patients, Sharon was delighted at the prospect of a better life. After she got on the program, she saw results in six weeks. "I used to feel awful, but now I feel better than I've felt in years!" she said. "My energy level is up and I'm doing more of the things I love to do. My husband used to ask, 'Don't you have something better to do other than just sit around?' Now he asks me if I would stay home with him for an evening. The Vitamin D Cure has made a world of difference for me."

Looking at Your Health Issues

Review the following list to see if you have any of these symptoms and/or diseases:

Symptoms

- Fatigue
- Joint pain and/or swelling
- Muscle pain, cramping, and/or weakness
- Chronic pain
- Uncontrolled weight gain
- High blood pressure
- Restless sleep
- Poor concentration and memory
- Headaches
- Bowel problems (constipation, diarrhea, or both)
- Bladder problems (urgency, frequency, or both)

Diseases

- Depression, including seasonal affective disorder (SAD)
- Fibromyalgia
- Parkinson's disease
- Alzheimer's disease
- Arthritis (osteoarthritis, gout, pseudogout, tendinitis, bursitis)
- Osteoporosis
- Gum disease and tooth loss
- Obesity
- Diabetes
- Heart disease
- Metabolic syndrome
- Autoimmune diseases (multiple sclerosis, systemic lupus erythematosis)
- Cancer

If you saw things on the preceding list that you deal with daily or weekly, get ready for some great news: all of these health problems (and many others) are related to vitamin D deficiency, and they can be helped by raising your vitamin D levels.

Your brain is first in line to detect the early symptoms of vitamin D deficiency, in the form of severe fatigue. Initially, you feel exhausted a lot of the time in late winter. The medical term for this is seasonal affective disorder (SAD) or seasonal depression.

But sometimes SAD persists. If suppressed D levels of wintertime were what led to your fatigue, the symptoms start piling up when the tiredness doesn't go away. Your mood sags, your sleep quality suffers, and the progression steadily worsens. Your behavior doesn't go unscathed, either. When you lose sleep and feel grouchy, you're not going to deliver stellar performances on a personal or a professional level.

At the same time, you're probably asking an obvious question: How do you know if you're just a little bit blue or grumpy or if you're really experiencing full-blown SAD? You can tell by two significant changes: reluctance to do any kind of physical activity, and a lack of enjoyment when you do things that used to please you.

A deflated attitude toward doing things is the first red flag. Doctors call it *psychomotor retardation,* a term for an overall lack of motivation to pursue activities that require you to be physical. The general thought process reflects a low mood.

A second red flag is a downward spiral in your general happiness level. Things you used to enjoy doing now simply sound like too much work. This is called *anhedonia,* and in some people this state can go on and on for years. You feel too bad to do anything, which makes you tired; you're tired, so you don't want to do anything. This vicious cycle can be endless if you fail to realize that a lack of vitamin D may be behind all your troubles.

You may have read that serotonin deficiency causes depression. Serotonin is a neurotransmitter (brain messenger) that affects your sense of well-being, and too little of it can make you feel depressed. You need sufficient serotonin to handle stress well and to feel content.

Recent research has focused on the role that brain inflammation plays in driving anhedonia, or the "blues," loss of motivation, and depression. Inflammation and stress appear to shift the conversion of the amino acid tryptophan away from important brain signal transmitters such as serotonin and melatonin, which improve mood and sleep, toward brain substances that promote anxiety and a depressed mood.

Vitamin D suppresses the activation of nuclear factors that trigger a cascade of inflammatory substances, including IL-6, tumor necrosis factor (TNF), interferon, and prostaglandins produced by white blood cells and certain brain cells. Inflammation is one way that vitamin D deficiency may aggravate the development of depression, seasonally and chronically, but vitamin D replacement addresses this problem.

Research tells us that a lack of vitamin D makes us ache. Symptoms that point to vitamin D deficiency are muscle spasms, bone pain, and joint pain.

When Mayo Clinic researchers looked at the vitamin D levels of patients who had unexplained widespread musculoskeletal pain for a long time, they found that 93 percent had vitamin D deficiency. Some of these people then took vitamin D and calcium supplements regularly, and the result was a dramatic resolution of their pain, fatigue, and muscle cramps.

Similarly, Dr. Al Faraj at Riyadh Armed Forces Hospital in Saudi Arabia discovered vitamin D deficiency in 83 percent of several hundred patients who had chronic back pain for more than six months without a diagnosis. When Dr. Faraj normalized the vitamin D of those with low vitamin D levels, the back pain resolved in all of them. Two-thirds of those with apparently normal vitamin D levels also eliminated back pain by taking D supplements.

If you're gaining weight and noting a general decline in your overall health, these changes probably indicate a lack of vitamin D, too. As you gain weight, your vitamin D level drops. These lower vitamin D levels in obesity are also associated with high blood pressure, poor glucose control, arthritis, and cancer.

Adequate vitamin D and the calcium it helps absorb may decrease the production of fat. Increased intake of vitamin D, calcium, and magnesium in the form of low-fat dairy products enhances weight loss along with calorie restriction. It appears that low calcium due to inadequate vitamin D or calcium in the diet triggers the release of the parathyroid hormone, which increases the concentration of activated vitamin D in fat cells and causes them to store energy as more fat.

Vitamin D affects your appetite as well. If you eat a high-calcium, high–vitamin D breakfast, you'll feel less hungry and probably eat less in the next twenty-four hours. A study that supports this theory looked at a group who consumed a breakfast low in calcium and vitamin D compared to a group who ate a breakfast high in calcium and vitamin D. The latter ate an average of three hundred fewer calories in the twenty-four hours following their breakfast.

Vitamin D Helps a Lot

Research keeps unearthing one finding after another that cites vitamin D deficiency as a major culprit in disease development. New studies show that vitamin D is important to proper brain development, and that a lack of this vitamin may be a contributing factor in causing schizophrenia, Parkinson's disease, and depression. Calcium and magnesium deficiencies often accompany vitamin D deficiency and are associated with seizures in infants and degenerative neurological disorders such as Parkinson's disease and Alzheimer's disease in adults.

The good news is that vitamin D

- relieves the symptoms of seasonal depression;
- plays a critical role in slowing or preventing many types of arthritis;
- reduces the likelihood that you'll have a heart attack or a stroke;
- improves the release of insulin and the response of muscle and liver to insulin, which means that normal levels of vitamin D may help prevent diabetes;

- helps you develop a healthy immune system during childhood; and

- plays a key role in regulating cell growth and differentiation, which may prevent cancer.

Shooting Down Myths

The following list shows the many discrepancies between research-based truths and the popular misconceptions that the media and some health-care providers continue to perpetuate.

By this point, you're probably excited about starting the Vitamin D Cure so you can get out of the D-deficiency danger zone. All you need do is follow the steps of the Vitamin D Cure program, and within about sixty days you'll feel loads better, look younger and trimmer, and be sprinting down the fast track to a lifetime of good health.

MYTHS AND TRUTHS

Vitamin D and Diet Myths	Vitamin D and Diet Truths
You can make an adequate amount of vitamin D with fifteen minutes of sun exposure three times a week or if you take 400 to 1,000 IU a day. Vitamin D daily requirements are the same for everyone regardless of size, age, and skin color.	You should supplement your vitamin D in a weight-based dose that you adjust according to your vitamin D blood level.
Normal vitamin D levels are above 20.	Normal vitamin D levels are above 30. Ideal vitamin D levels are between 40 and 60.
Adults need 1,200 milligrams of calcium a day, and postmenopausal women and adults sixty-five or older need 1,500 milligrams a day.	You will not need any additional calcium in the form of supplements if your diet is acid base–balanced and your vitamin D levels are between 40 and 60.
Osteoporosis is a disease of aging that begins after menopause.	Osteoporosis is a disease that begins before birth and in childhood with vitamin D deficiency, dietary imbalance, and lack of exercise. The failure to attain peak bone mass in early adult life leads to osteoporosis as an older adult.

Vitamin D and Diet Myths	Vitamin D and Diet Truths
Vitamin D and excess calcium cause kidney stones.	Kidney stones are due to acid excess in our diet that translates into acidic urine, which is high in calcium and primed for stone formation. The cause is not eating enough green vegetables.
The USDA promoted "The Food Pyramid," then "My Pyramid," and now "My Plate," with roughly the same 5–8 ounces of grain and 3 cups of dairy a day. It equates beans to meat and says that you should have 5–6 ounces of protein a day.	This is too much acid, too many calories, and too little lean protein and green veggies. Animal protein provides more satisfaction than grains, cheese, or beans because it has two to four times more protein per serving.
Obesity is simply taking in too many calories and not burning enough calories.	Obesity is a disease of inadequate nutrition. We eat until we satisfy our nutritional needs (hunger). With lean meat and fresh produce, we can do this in smaller caloric packages than with grains and dairy.
Following a very-low-calorie diet is the fastest and healthiest way to lose weight.	When you starve yourself to a lower weight, you lose fat, bone, and muscle in the process. Increasing lean fat-burning muscle mass is essential to fitness. When you exercise to lose fat and lose weight, you also gain muscle and bone.
Osteoarthritis is a disease of age and wear-and-tear.	Osteoarthritis is a disease of bone remodeling caused by vitamin D deficiency and dietary acid excess.
Autoimmune diseases are primarily genetic disorders.	Autoimmune diseases are due to genetic risk in the presence of vitamin D deficiency and dietary imbalance beginning shortly after conception and continuing through early childhood.
Cancer is due to genetics and sometimes environmental carcinogens.	Cancer is usually a preventable disease if you have a lifetime of normal vitamin D levels and a healthy diet.

(continued)

MYTHS AND TRUTHS *(continued)*

Vitamin D and Diet Myths	Vitamin D and Diet Truths
Melanoma results from too much sun exposure.	Melanoma results from overexposure to UVA and inadequate vitamin D levels.
It isn't cost-effective to screen everybody for vitamin D deficiency.	Vitamin D should be measured at routine physical examinations for people of all ages.

2

How Vitamin D Works

Vitamin D deficiency is

- more common in women;
- more common in people of color;
- more common in obese people;
- more common as you get older; and
- more common in breast-fed infants.

Marianna complained of constant pain; she told her family and friends she was always "dead tired." She knew little about vitamin D, but she was acutely aware of feeling bad most of the time.

"When Dr. Dowd first introduced me to his vitamin D program, I was skeptical because I'd seen lots of doctors who weren't able to help me, and I found it hard to believe the solution could be so simple," Marianna said. "But within two weeks of taking vitamin D supplements and changing my diet, the fatigue I'd had for years began melting away. Now I have the energy to exercise again. I don't wake up exhausted or in pain, and I don't go to bed every night hurting."

Understanding vitamin D can help you recognize why your symptoms and diseases are worse when you're deficient in vitamin D. It also can help you use the great health potential of vitamin D. An understanding of how vitamin D can help you get well will be critical in motivating you to make a few lifestyle changes. Let's get acquainted with this important fat-soluble vitamin that comes from cholesterol.

Despite its name, vitamin D isn't actually a vitamin. Vitamins are organic substances you get from dietary sources; vitamin D is produced by your body. When your skin is exposed to UVB (ultraviolet B) radiation from the sun, pre-vitamin D is modified. Next, this fat-soluble pre-vitamin is transported to the liver and the kidneys, where it's converted into the forms your tissues require. It becomes *activated vitamin D*, which fits its name because it has now turned into an active participant in your bodily processes.

Pre-vitamin D is made in the liver, and ultraviolet B sunlight plus heat twist the pre-vitamin D in a reaction that forms vitamin D_3 in the skin. When it's further activated in the liver and again in the kidneys and other tissues, it turns into a potent hormone. You can't make any of the active forms of vitamin D without the UVB step.

Many forms of active vitamin D exist—some are more potent than others—and they all serve slightly different cell functions. A mixture of different forms of vitamin D is what's doing the work in your body. Your own physical and biochemical demands and your supply of vitamin D from sunlight or supplementation determine the composition of this mixture.

Two forms of vitamin D that we examine in this book are the vitamin D you make with sunlight or take in the form of supplements and activated vitamin D. Your body's actual supply of vitamin D determines in large part how much activated vitamin D you can make. Keep in mind that activated vitamin D is the potent hormone that does most of the work.

We use the terms "vitamin D" and "activated vitamin D" interchangeably. We don't advocate taking the prescription form of activated D (calcitriol) as part of the Vitamin D Cure.

It's important to know that activated vitamin D is made for both systemic (whole-body) and local purposes. It's like the way that computer software comes with updates and technical support; the support is global, as well as individual. You automatically get updates for your software, and so does everyone else who has the same software. But if you have a specific problem, you can request specific support.

By the same token, you need a certain amount of activated vitamin D circulating throughout your body, and your kidneys are responsible for that task. You may, however, need extra-activated vitamin D for specific local needs, such as an infection in your lungs or cancer cells in your breast. The cells in your lungs and breast are able to make that extra amount of activated vitamin D as long as you have a big enough supply of vitamin D from the sun or supplements. If you don't, you're out of luck, because your body can't deal with the local threat as effectively.

Properties of Vitamin D

Vitamin D is a unique hormone that belongs to a group called the steroid hormone family. All of the hormones in this family are made from cholesterol, and they include cortisol, estrogen, progesterone, and testosterone.

This family is known for developing partnerships with other hormones. They all bind to nuclear receptors, meaning they have access to the nucleus, where they influence gene expression. Some of vitamin D's favorite partnerships are with vitamin A, thyroid hormone, and variations of growth hormone. These relationships help define the function of vitamin D in different situations. Probably vitamin D's most important partnership is the one with vitamin A or other molecules, such as omega-3 fats that bind to the vitamin A receptor.

When vitamin D binds to its receptor, it almost always does so in partnership with the vitamin A receptor, which binds vitamin A or the omega-3 fatty acid DHA. In the nucleus of the cell, it sits as judge and jury, deciding which genes are turned on and which are turned off.

We aren't just talking a seat on the front row—vitamin D and its partners vitamin A and DHA are conducting the orchestra.

Most people know that vitamin D is important in helping our body to absorb calcium from food. D's importance in the formation of bone and teeth in children is also widely known. In addition, vitamin D helps you build muscle and protects your brain cells from injury or inflammation.

Vitamin D slows the growth of cells—a factor that may well reduce your risk of some cancers by as much as 50 percent. Vitamin D is also crucial for fertility, glucose control, reducing high blood pressure, and ameliorating seasonal affective disorder. Vitamin D helps you fight infections and improves the effectiveness of vaccines. Without enough vitamin D, your risk of autoimmune diseases may increase by as much as 300 percent.

The Sun and Vitamin D

Most people mistakenly think that they get enough vitamin D from casual sun exposure or their diets. Unfortunately, this is not true. People in today's urban digital society rarely get enough sun exposure to fill their vitamin D requirement, and nondietary sources must meet about 90 percent of your daily D needs.

The more melanin you have in your skin and the faster you tan, the more sunlight you need to convert pre-vitamin D to vitamin D you can use. The melanin in your skin acts as a natural sunscreen that blocks up to 90 percent of UV light. Dark African Americans need about seven times as much sunlight as fair-skinned European Americans to manufacture the necessary amount of vitamin D.

When equatorial dwellers immigrate to the United States, they move from overexposure at the equator, and their melanin, which once provided protection from the sun, now turns into a handicap in making vitamin D. This is a major reason for African Americans' higher incidence of obesity, high blood pressure, diabetes, gout, heart disease, systemic lupus, and cancer.

You may be thinking, I just need to take this book to my doctor and ask for a prescription to move to Florida or Southern California so I can get enough sunshine.

That's not the solution, and here's why: you have to live a lifestyle that lets you get outside to soak up sunlight. If your lifestyle doesn't allow that, you could live in Hawaii and be D deficient.

You won't see much difference in the D levels of people living in Florida and those from the northern United States, simply because culture, urbanization, and technology have lured all of us indoors and out of the sun during the last quarter century. Moreover, the smog in large metropolitan areas decreases D production, compared to rural areas at the same latitude.

The casual sunlight exposure of today's urban lifestyle isn't enough to produce adequate amounts of vitamin D, no matter what your latitude. That's why the Vitamin D Cure is essential!

3

The Diet–Vitamin D Connection

The vitamin D deficiency picture is a bit more complicated than it seems on the surface. You can correct your vitamin D levels and help yourself immensely with that one easy upgrade. But you can really do worlds of good for your health by taking into account the other missing ingredients in your diet—and fixing those, too.

If you eat like many North Americans, you probably have these faux pas to correct:

- You eat too many grains and cheese, which are acid-producing.
- You don't get enough magnesium-rich foods.
- You don't get enough potassium-rich foods.

Neutralizing the Acid

The more acid you produce, the more potassium, magnesium, and calcium you need to buffer the acid. The potential effects of too much acid on your body are a bit scary. Failure to eat enough antacid-producing fruits and vegetables high in potassium, magnesium, and calcium means that you end up borrowing from your body's vault of minerals and protein in your bones, muscles, and joints.

Here's how it works: everything you eat is metabolized in the liver, where your body extracts energy and nutrition and produces waste products that are eliminated as urine. Waste is acidic, neutral, or alkaline (antacid), depending on the type of nutrient. Protein leads to acid waste, and vegetables and fruits lead to alkaline or antacid waste.

Remember that we're talking about waste, not taste. Lemons, oranges, and tomatoes contain antacid, not acid; these are good guys because they're loaded with potassium and magnesium citrate and they generate bicarbonate, which serves as a buffer when metabolized.

On the other hand, think of table salt as a hole in your nutrition vault. You eat veggies and fruits to pack your vault with potassium, magnesium, and calcium, but the sodium chloride you eat zaps your potassium, magnesium, and calcium—and then urine exiles the good minerals.

Lean meat, including seafood, pork tenderloin, skinless chicken breast, and skinless turkey breast, produces about 9 points (milliequivalents or mEq) of acid per 3.5-ounce serving. Nuts and whole grains give you about 7 points of acid per equivalent serving; bread and legumes, about half that.

Cheese, however, produces on average *20 points of acid* per serving—two to three times more acid than other protein sources. Cheese also is loaded with salt and saturated fat. This is the dairy industry's dirty little secret: tell Americans to eat three servings of dairy a day, but don't tell them to avoid cheese. The truth is, cheese has no redeeming qualities; I call it the king of junk food. Unfortunately, cheese is the only dairy product with growing sales.

The average American diet contains about 30 to 50 points of excess acid a day. How quickly you can discard this acid in your urine depends on how well hydrated you are and how much kidney function you have. The older you are, the less acid you can handle because your kidney function declines with age. If you have long-standing diabetes or high blood pressure, these diseases reduce your kidney function and your capacity to dump acid. If you're dehydrated because you're not drinking enough water or eating enough fluid-filled fruits and veggies, you are stuck with acid. If you're on "water pills," these will not only dehydrate you, they will also cause you to waste excessive amounts of potassium and magnesium, both of which may aggravate the acid excess.

Acid excess (acidosis) is a stress on your system. Your body undergoes a stress response in an effort to neutralize the imbalance. The changes include higher cortisol levels; lower growth hormone levels; and higher renin, angiotensin, and aldosterone levels.

Such changes hurt your health. They decrease your bone and muscle mass by withdrawing potassium, magnesium, calcium, and protein from your bones. They increase abdominal fat stores, which lowers available vitamin D and produces more inflammatory substances. These changes raise your blood pressure and increase the loss of potassium and magnesium in your urine. This renders your remaining vitamin D less effective.

The key consequences of this stress response to acidosis are:

- Increased abdominal fat
- Insulin resistance
- Increased production of inflammatory substances
- Mobilization of bone and muscle as buffers

These lead to the *metabolic syndrome*, which carries an increased risk of heart disease, stroke, and diabetes.

Why You Need Magnesium, Too

If you don't have enough magnesium to jump-start your bodily functions, you won't be able to produce the activated form of vitamin D and energize it to do its business of gene regulation. Lacking the proper amount of magnesium, you may become resistant to vitamin D.

Magnesium is so important that without it, we would cease to exist. Magnesium is required for chlorophyll to function properly; chlorophyll is the green pigment in plants that's necessary for photosynthesis. No magnesium, no plant life. We humans need magnesium for more than three hundred enzymatic reactions, bone formation, and muscle and nerve function, in addition to the job of buffering acid waste from protein digestion.

Here are some problems you may suffer if you have insufficient magnesium:

- Your body will have more trouble converting vitamin D to the activated vitamin D that your body can actually use.

- You won't be able to produce and use the important energy unit ATP.

- Your body won't work as well because low magnesium decreases expression of vitamin D receptors and impairs receptor signaling.

- Your body won't be able to use very well what calcium and magnesium you have. Low magnesium suppresses the release of parathyroid hormone (PTH) and calcitonin, hormones that help regulate the metabolism of calcium and magnesium.

- You compromise the activity of enzymes that regulate your membrane mineral pumps. Like levee pumps, your body's membrane mineral pumps keep potassium inside the cell and sodium outside the cell, as well as performing other functions.

- Your body loses much-needed potassium and calcium via your urine.

How to Get Enough Magnesium and Potassium

Magnesium is an antacid. You need the antacids in your body—potassium, magnesium, and calcium—to neutralize acid waste. The more antacids you consume in your diet, the fewer you have to borrow from your body stores. And the more protein you eat, the more antacid you need to buffer the acid waste that comes from digesting protein.

To get enough magnesium so your vitamin D functions properly, and to facilitate those all-important enzymatic reactions, you must

- eat a magnesium-rich diet; and
- balance the acid-base in your diet to reduce loss of magnesium (and other buffers) in urine.

You can get plenty of magnesium from vegetables and fruits, particularly green, leafy, chlorophyll-rich vegetables such as spinach, bok choy, kale, collard greens, and Swiss chard. Nuts are also great for beefing up your magnesium. Whole grains contain lots of magnesium, but the downside is that they also have phytates that reduce absorption of magnesium. Moreover, whole grains and nuts generate acid when metabolized, whereas vegetables and fruits generate antacid. Fresh produce is better than grains and nuts for getting and holding on to magnesium.

If you eat a typical North American diet, you probably consume two servings of produce a day—and you eat fruit more often than you eat green, leafy vegetables. But you probably get only about 60 percent of the amount of magnesium the CDC tells us we need.

According to the National Academy of Sciences, an adult needs about 2.7 milligrams per pound of lean body weight (2.3 milligrams per pound for children). That means that if you're 150 pounds and lean, for example, you need 420 milligrams of magnesium a day.

Unfortunately, popping a magnesium supplement isn't the perfect answer because your body doesn't absorb these supplements very well: absorption efficiency from magnesium supplements can be as low as 5 to 15 percent. Another problem with magnesium supplements is that they can give you diarrhea. This side effect is obnoxious enough to limit your interest in relying on magnesium supplements for your dietary magnesium.

On the other hand, you absorb 25 to 50 percent of the magnesium in foods. You need to get most of your magnesium from your diet. Spinach, bok choy, kale, and Swiss chard will give you as much as five times more magnesium than supplements. Green, leafy vegetables are a real nutrition bargain because you get magnesium as well as calcium, potassium, trace minerals, antacids, vitamin K, polyphenols, antioxidants, and fiber.

If you take blood thinners that are affected by the vitamin K in green, leafy vegetables, you'll need to take magnesium supplements. For someone on blood thinners, it's more important to eat a consistent amount of green, leafy vegetables than to avoid them altogether. It is the variability in green, leafy vegetables/vitamin K intake that throws off the dosing of your blood thinners.

Water pills (diuretics) will make you lose excessive amounts of potassium and magnesium in your urine, so if you're on water pills, be sure to take supplements as part of your daily regimen.

As for potassium, most people need to double the amount they typically consume. So try to increase your intake of potassium-rich foods—vegetables, fruits, and nuts. Try these quick tips:

- Make a habit of consuming a handful of nuts (ten to twelve) each day.
- Fill your fruit bowl with bananas, which will help you remember to eat one a day.
- Don't eat cheese.
- Seldom eat grains.
- Consume lots of green, leafy vegetables and fruits that are rich in magnesium and potassium.
- Don't add salt to your foods, and avoid presalted foods.

Next, we'll move on to the Vitamin D Cure Five-Step Plan.

The Vitamin D Cure Five-Step Plan

Part two gets down to the heart of the Vitamin D Cure. We show you how you can help yourself by following the five steps of the Vitamin D Cure.

1. Find out how much vitamin D you need.
2. Sun and supplement your way to great D levels.
3. Reduce your acid excess by changing your diet.
4. Cover your bases with other supplements.
5. Add a little exercise.

This program can literally give you a new lease on good health, but first find out if you actually need more vitamin D. Most people do, but you won't know for sure until you take the quiz in chapter 4 or have your doctor do a blood test that shows your vitamin D level.

If you discover that you're D deficient, like most North Americans, proceed to the rest of the steps. You will get started on the right amount of vitamin D supplementation for your weight. Examine your diet for acid-base imbalance, and then make specific moves to ensure the balance that can ward off diseases.

You also want to make sure that your supplementation regimen includes all the vitamins you need, and chapter 7 helps you get that action under way. Finally, add in some very simple moves that won't take up much time but are super underpinnings for the Vitamin D Cure; you'll maximize your results by adding a simple exercise regimen.

Follow the steps and face every day with renewed optimism, energy, and excitement. When you realize it doesn't take much more than eating better foods and taking vitamin D supplements, this is a truly simple path to renewed health!

4

Step One: Find Out How Much Vitamin D You Need

First, figure out where you stand. Start with an assessment of your need for vitamin D:

- Take the quiz below.

- See a physician if you want guidance in assessing your vitamin D.

- Get the right tests if you need testing. (This isn't a requirement, though, because you can definitely start the Vitamin D Cure without taking blood tests.)

- Figure out what your test results mean in regard to your overall health.

If you wish to follow up on your vitamin D level, you can check to see if your supplements are on target after you've been on supplements for a few months.

Vitamin D Risk Analysis Quiz

☐ Your ethnic background is half or more than half African, Indian, Southeast Asian, Latin American, or Arabic (or if you have skin type 4, 5, or 6—see the Sun Exposure Times chart in chapter 5 on page 46). (3 points)

☐ Your body mass index (BMI) is 30 or greater. (3 points) See page 116 to calculate your BMI.

☐ You are a breast-fed infant who is not on vitamin or formula supplements. (3 points)

☐ You have fatigue or recurring muscle, bone, or joint pain. (2 points)

☐ You are fifty years or older. (2 points)

☐ You live outside the thirty-fifth parallel north or south of the equator. (2 points) See the map below.

☐ You wear sunscreen of SPF 8 or greater before you go outdoors. (2 points)

☐ You rarely (fewer than three times a week) spend time outdoors between 11:00 a.m. and 4:00 p.m. (2 points)

☐ You are a woman (1 point)

☐ _____ *Total score*

Scoring for each section:

0–2 points	Low risk
3–5 points	High risk
> 5 points	Very high risk

You can go online to take your Vitamin D Risk Analysis Quiz—www.thevitamindcure.com.

If your score shows that you're high risk or very high risk, you need to increase your vitamin D production with sun or supplements (see chapter 5). If you're in the low-risk group, you may want to consider having your vitamin D level measured. (I measure every patient so I can customize treatment to each individual.)

Some people, however, prefer to skip blood tests and proceed straight to vitamin D supplementation. This is perfectly acceptable, but it leaves you guessing why you may or may not have responded the way you expected.

United States Latitude Map

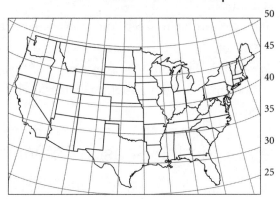

If you're not feeling better in two months or if you just want to know where you stand, you may want to go to your doctor to get tested. See "The Right Vitamin D Tests" beginning on page 229 for more information.

Keep Your D Level Above Thirty-Something

Evidence points to 30 ng/mL (75 nmol/L) as the lower limit of normal vitamin D. Even at a microscopic level, the bone mineral defect diseases rickets and osteomalacia don't occur in a person with adequate vitamin D levels.

In a 2010 German study on the bone composition of healthy adults who died in accidents, scientists found that bone mineralization was never abnormal in individuals with a vitamin D level higher than 30. The farther the vitamin D level was below this threshold, though, the more common abnormal mineralization of bone was.

In people who have a vitamin D level of less than 30, the risk of type 2 diabetes, colon cancer, cardiovascular events, and death from all causes rises dramatically. Furthermore, your absorption of dietary calcium is impaired if your D level is lower than 35.

A University of Colorado study published in 2011 showed that at a vitamin D level of about 40, the parathyroid gland begins to secrete more of its hormone to activate vitamin D and pull calcium out of the bones. This means that when your D level is between 30 and 40, your body begins to compensate, and when your level drops below 30, it goes into full disaster mode.

To ward off health problems, keep your D level higher than 30 and, ideally, between 40 and 60. This is consistent with studies of lifeguards and farmers in equatorial regions who spend most of their days in the sun. It's better to overshoot with a slightly higher level than risk dire health consequences.

Understanding the Seasons of Vitamin D

Immigration to the United States and migration within America, from rural agricultural centers in the South to industrial cities in the Northeast and Midwest, have led to decreased sun exposure for millions of Americans. For example, when you move north from the lower Mississippi or Gulf Coast to Detroit, Michigan, you have 40 to 50 percent fewer days for vitamin D production. Combine that with a 75 percent decrease in sun exposure when you leave outdoor jobs to work inside and you have a virtual vitamin D crisis.

Because vitamin D levels fluctuate with varying sun exposure, yours are probably highest at the end of summer (September to October) and lowest at the end of winter (February to April). The farther you move from the equator, the greater these fluctuations. Although you don't have to measure your vitamin D level, the ideal time of year to do this if you want to detect your deficiency is at winter's end, because that's when you'll get your lowest value for the year.

But if you're concerned about vitamin D–related health troubles right now, don't wait to measure your level. Start the program. You can always measure your D level later to see if your supplementation is on target. At that time you may decide you want to measure your peak and trough to see if your levels fall within the 40–60 range.

Seasons of the Sun

In the following illustration, you can see the seasonal fluctuations of vitamin D blood levels. People living in nursing homes who get little or no sun exposure may not have significant changes in vitamin D from one

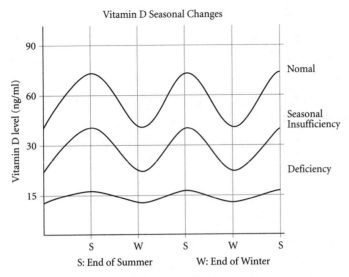

Vitamin D Seasonal Changes

This figure represents the relationship between vitamin D and the seasons. A person is deficient if he or she gets little or no sun and has vitamin D levels that change very little with the seasons. Someone who has a great deal of skin melanin experiences a downward shift in the vitamin D curve and a blunting of seasonal fluctuations in vitamin D.

season to the next. On the other hand, farmers in Minnesota may be outdoors most of the time during spring and summer, but they live so far north their bodies can't make adequate vitamin D from October through April. If you're a Minnesota farmer whose vitamin D level is 40 in September, that figure will drop to 20 by January and may decline by 50 percent again by early spring, leaving you extremely D deficient. Similarly, submarine sailors lose about 50 percent of their vitamin D after they go without UVB light for ten weeks.

What's the best way to enhance your vitamin D level? Number one: get more sun exposure. It sounds simple, but it's really not that simple, because you can get enough sun exposure only if you spend lots of time outside *and* you live in a place where there's a UV index of 3 or higher. Here's how the National Oceanic and Atmospheric Administration (NOAA) explains the UV index:

> The annual UV index is a graphical report of the amount of skin-damaging UV radiation expected to reach the earth's surface at the time when the sun is highest in the sky (solar noon). The amount of UV radiation reaching the surface is primarily related to

the elevation of the sun in the sky, the amount of ozone in the stratosphere, and the amount of clouds present. The UV index can range from 0 (nighttime) to 15 or 16 (in the tropics at high elevations under clear skies). UV radiation is greatest when the sun is highest in the sky and rapidly decreases as the sun approaches the horizon. The higher the UV index, the greater the dose rate of skin-damaging (and eye-damaging) UV radiation. Consequently, the higher the UV index, the less time it takes before skin damage occurs.

The UV index is not solely a measure of UVB light, but UVB plays the largest role in calculating the UV index. And because the UV index is available throughout the year, it's a useful tool for estimating your capacity to make vitamin D.

To make any vitamin D, you need a UV index of about 3 or greater. The higher the UV index, the shorter the time you need to make an adequate amount of vitamin D. See chapter 5 for a chart that shows how to calculate your sun exposure needs.

You can locate your annual UV index report by city at the following Web site: www.cpc.ncep.noaa.gov/products/stratosphere/uv_index/uv_annual.shtml.

Note that the lower line on the daily UV index plot takes into account cloud cover and how it suppresses UV index. In a place such as Michigan, that means lots of days with a lower UV index.

To get your calculated UV index, check www.epa.gov/sunwise/uvindex.html or weather underground online, www.wunderground.com. Your current forecasted UV index will appear under "Current Data—Health." See the following illustration for the differences between Detroit, Michigan, and Houston, Texas.

You can see that the number of days with a moderate or higher UV index in Detroit is 180, compared to 299 per year in Houston. That translates to 40 percent fewer days available for making vitamin D.

Looking at this in yet another way, we know that you can make vitamin D only from April 15 to September 30 in Detroit. That's just 5½ months. But the reality is that few working people take outdoor lunch breaks, and many work five or six days a week. That basically leaves

Daily UV Index

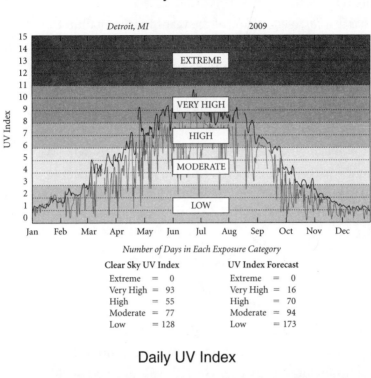

Detroit, MI   2009

Number of Days in Each Exposure Category

Clear Sky UV Index			UV Index Forecast		
Extreme	=	0	Extreme	=	0
Very High	=	93	Very High	=	16
High	=	55	High	=	70
Moderate	=	77	Moderate	=	94
Low	=	128	Low	=	173

Daily UV Index

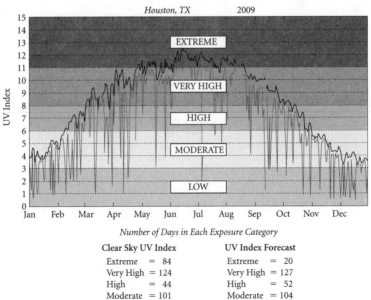

Houston, TX   2009

Number of Days in Each Exposure Category

Clear Sky UV Index			UV Index Forecast		
Extreme	=	84	Extreme	=	20
Very High	=	124	Very High	=	127
High	=	44	High	=	52
Moderate	=	101	Moderate	=	104
Low	=	0	Low	=	50

weekends from May to September, because it's usually still too cold in April to expose much skin. This means that someone who lives in Michigan has just *forty-eight days* of the year to make vitamin D.

Locale isn't the only stumbling block to D production. Sunscreen with an SPF as low as 8 blocks almost 98 percent of UVB rays, which makes it practically impossible to make vitamin D if you wear sunscreen.

Where you sit or stand matters, too. You can't make vitamin D sitting next to a window in your home, your office, and your car because most modern glass technology blocks most UVB light. Wear a wide-brimmed hat and long sleeves, and you get no D either.

If casual sun exposure is defined as fifteen minutes of sun (see Q&A on page 207), three times a week year round, let's see how that fits into forty-eight days.

15 minutes/day × 3 days/week × 52 weeks/year
= 2,340 minutes/48 days
= 49 minutes/day

About fifty minutes of sun exposure on each of the forty-eight days available may allow you to produce enough vitamin D. But how safe is that amount of sun twice a week if you get no sun for five to six months? Can you store up enough D during forty-eight days to last for the six months when you can't make vitamin D in Michigan?

Based on varying amounts of sun exposure, vitamin D levels fluctuate from their high at the end of summer (September to October) to their low at the end of winter (March to April). The farther you move from the equator, the greater these fluctuations. Diet contributes very little to seasonal fluctuations in vitamin D levels.

If you're using blood work to gauge your supplementation, measure your vitamin D level every three months and make adjustments until it fluctuates between 40 and 60. You want your vitamin D level to stay above 30 all the time.

Why the Vitamin D Cure Works

When can you expect to feel better? Some people notice an increase in energy and a decrease in pain only two weeks into the program. Typically, though, it takes about two and a half to three months to bring your vitamin D level up to a new plateau.

More than half the people who are deficient in vitamin D also lack magnesium—and vitamin D won't work very well without adequate magnesium in place. To complete the vitamin D supplementation package, you must make the necessary dietary changes and/or take the right supplements to restore normal magnesium levels.

Magnesium restoration, unlike the vitamin D upgrade, can take many months. The problem is, you can't accurately assess your magnesium status very easily with commonly available blood tests. If you're assessing your magnesium level, you'll get more information from a written analysis of your eating patterns than you will from blood tests. Furthermore, the movement of magnesium between storage compartments (blood, inside cells, bone) is very slow. Replenishing bone with magnesium may take a year.

As you continue the program, you'll see even more improvements in your health for years because bone remodeling and replenishment of long-term stores of magnesium and calcium can take months to years.

Finding Your Yardstick

Medicine likes using standardized tools to measure progress in a treatment program. For ten years, my clinic has used a validated tool to assess the visit-to-visit progress of my patients on the Vitamin D Cure program. The tool—the Clinical Modified Health Assessment Questionnaire II (CLINHAQII)—is a series of questions and scales that people complete while in the waiting room each time they come in for an office visit. Clinic staffers score these patients and enter the information into a flow sheet in their charts.

This tool assigns an objective or measurable number to a patient's symptoms so we can make comparisons and note progress from one month to the next. We use 16 questions to score ease of daily activities and rate certain areas in the following ways:

1. *Help or no help?* To accomplish a certain activity, do you need no assistance, some assistance, or a great deal? Or are you unable to

complete the activity? A 0 means you can perform all the activities questioned with no assistance (no help, canes, or walkers). A 3 means you're completely dependent on others for help in performing an activity; you can't complete the task on your own.

2. *Pain or no pain?* Rate pain via a visual scale (0–100); 0 is no pain, and 100 represents the worst pain you have ever experienced.

3. *Fatigue or no fatigue?* This puts a number on fatigue (0–100); 0 means no fatigue at all, and 100 stands for the worst fatigue ever.

4. *Healthy or not healthy?* The fourth number in the series is a visual scale for perception of overall health; 0 means no health problems at all; 100 means that this individual rates his or her overall health as awful.

5. *Restful sleep or sleep problems?* Zero means you have no restful sleep; 10 is very restful sleep.

You'll find the latest CLINHAQII test at National Databank for Rheumatic diseases (www.arthritis-research.org/); just click on the "Clinic/Research" tab and open the "Questionnaires" file.

What the Numbers Mean

A patient with a CLINHAQII series of 0.5–80–100–65–4 has the following symptoms:

- 0.5/100 assistance to move—she needs little assistance.
- 80/100 pain—she is in a lot of pain.
- 100/100 fatigue—she's very tired all the time.
- 65/100 health perception—she doesn't feel well overall.
- 4/10 sleep—she's not getting restful sleep.

This person was pretty miserable. She began supplementation, came back to my office, and her new scores were 0–20–20–10–7. This says:

- She never needs assistance to move.
- Her relief from pain improved 75 percent.

- She feels more energetic—her fatigue has improved 80 percent, dropping from 100 to 20.
- She feels 85 percent better—she's experiencing much more restful sleep.

Now let's look at some people who followed the Vitamin D Cure at the Arthritis Institute of Michigan.

MARTA'S STIFFNESS

One doctor thought Marta, fifty-three, had fibromyalgia; another physician's diagnosis was rheumatoid arthritis. She wanted a treatment plan, so she came to see us at the Arthritis Institute of Michigan.

Marta had pain and swelling in her fingers. The problem had gone on for two months, gradually getting worse. Now and then she also had pain and stiffness in her hips, knees, feet, and shoulders. She had high blood pressure, episodes of depression, and frequent constipation. I saw some bony enlargement of her knuckles that was consistent with osteoarthritis in her hands. Her muscles, shins, and bones were tender. Overall, though, she was in good health.

Her initial CLINHAQII score was 0.375–65–70–70–5 (function, pain, fatigue, health perception, sleep). Lab tests revealed normal thyroid and rheumatoid factors but a slightly elevated C-reactive protein (a measure of inflammation). Her vitamin D level, though, was only 12 despite normal parathyroid hormone (PTH) and calcium.

Marta started vitamin D of 38 IU per pound per day. I advised her to follow these diet rules:

- Avoid salt, cheese, and grains.
- Eat fresh produce and lean protein in a 3:1 ratio.

She improved her diet, took supplements, and when we saw her three months later, she posted great results. Her scores were 0.25–35–25–25–9, and her stiffness had gone from an all-day event to two hours per day. At her six-month follow-up visit, she scored

0.25–25–25–15–8 and reported only one hour of morning stiffness. Her relief from pain had improved by more than 60 percent, her fatigue by more than 60 percent, and her sleep quality by 70 percent.

Doctors often mistake vitamin D and dietary deficiencies for fibromyalgia, rheumatoid arthritis, and lupus. This shows how important it is to make sure your doctor checks your vitamin D level and diet if you're trying to find answers for long-term fatigue and persistent muscle and bone pain. By the same token, people who have rheumatoid arthritis, lupus, and/or fibromyalgia also may have vitamin D and dietary deficiencies, so this is tricky to diagnose.

KATIE'S ACHES, FATIGUE, IRRITABLE BOWEL SYNDROME, AND POOR SLEEP

Katie, thirty-five, ached all over. She was going to have surgery to relieve her foot pain. Her health problems included disc disease in her lower back and neck, polycystic ovarian disease, headaches, depression, and irritable bowel syndrome. For six years, the pain had been getting worse. She was having muscle twitching and cramps, swollen and stiff fingers, sleep disturbances, and generalized muscle and bone tenderness. Her shins and the tops of her feet hurt.

Lab studies revealed very slight inflammation but normal general chemistries, blood counts, rheumatoid factor tests, and antinuclear antibody tests. Her CLINHAQII scores were 0.75–80–40–50–5 (function, pain, fatigue, health perception, sleep), and she said she felt stiff for about 30 minutes in the morning. Her weight was 199 pounds. Her vitamin D level was 14, with a PTH of 58 and normal calcium.

We started her on vitamin D 25 IU per pound per day and calcium and magnesium supplements. She began avoiding salt, cheese, and grains and ate more fresh produce and lean protein.

Three months later, with a new vitamin D level of 48, Katie had lowered her CLINHAQII scores to 0–0–35–25–7. She now had only a couple of minutes of stiffness in the morning; her weight was 196 pounds. She was functioning normally, and most of her pain had disappeared. She slept better, and the stiffness had resolved. Overall, she felt 50 percent better.

Six months into the program, with a D level of 70 at the end of summer, Katie scored 0–0–20–0–6. She weighed 189 pounds; her function was normal; and she had no pain. She had less stomach pain, constipation, and diarrhea. Overall, she felt 100 percent better once she was taking vitamin D 25 IU per pound per day. Polycystic ovarian disease is a condition related to diabetes and obesity in women and is often associated with infertility. In many such people, vitamin D replacement restores fertility.

MARTIN'S PAIN

We saw an eleven-year-old African American boy, Martin, who had a three-year history of pain in his legs, arms, hands, ankles, and feet, with no swelling. He had worse pain in the winter but felt better in the summer (he spent summers in Mississippi). His muscles and bones hurt, especially in the shins, but he was healthy overall.

Martin had CLINHAQII scores of 0.875–50–50–70–7 (function, pain, fatigue, health perception, sleep); in the morning, he felt stiff for about half an hour. Lab tests revealed a vitamin D level of 11, normal PTH, and normal calcium. Blood counts were normal; one inflammatory test was slightly elevated.

We put Martin on vitamin D of 45 IU per pound per day, and after three months his CLINHAQII scores were 0–30–20–30–9, and his vitamin D level was 25, even though he'd been taking vitamin D inconsistently. He no longer felt stiff.

After six months on the program, with more consistent vitamin D intake, Martin posted scores of 0–0–0–5–9. His vitamin D level was 35 on vitamin D 40 IU per pound. This shows that people continue to experience improvements for six or more months into the program.

African Americans of all ages have at least a 90 percent chance of having vitamin D deficiency. Family members often share the same lifestyle and eating habits, so they often have the same vitamin D and dietary deficiencies. Martin's mother realized that she, too, was deficient in vitamin D, so she began taking supplements.

5

Step Two: Sun and Supplement Your Way to Great D Levels

Step Two of the Vitamin D Cure is the most important: Replenish your vitamin D with sun and supplements. Here's how:

- Maximize your safe sun exposure.
- Use sunscreen only after you have gotten your fill of vitamin D.
- Take vitamin D (you can figure out the proper dose after reading your risk score and/or your blood level figures).
- Don't forget that children need vitamin D more than you do.
- Stay away from too much vitamin A when you are supplementing with vitamin D.

GEORGIA'S STORY

The way the Vitamin D Cure solves problems is abundantly clear in many people, and one great example that comes to mind is Georgia, a fifty-seven-year-old woman I first saw five years ago in my office at the Arthritis Institute of Michigan. At the time she was suffering from numerous health problems, including a history of migraine headaches, which had backed off somewhat since she'd gone through menopause.

A bigger menace, though, was her long-standing history of fatigue and pain in her shoulders, back, and hips. Bouts of restless sleep made her even more exhausted. Neck and shoulder pain sometimes limited her mobility. Her hip pain got worse with prolonged sitting; walking also was painful. Georgia had muscle cramps in her legs and feet. Even pain medications and physical therapy hadn't helped.

Two decades earlier, Georgia had reported depression; her doctor thought this problem was probably a spin-off of her divorce. Ten years later, with a new diagnosis of fibromyalgia, she sought help at a pain management center. Several medications and injections later, though, Georgia was still in pain, but as she put it, "I decided I'd just live with my problems. I don't like to take drugs because they cloud my thinking."

But her poor health didn't let up. Fifteen years ago, a doctor discovered decreased thyroid function and put her on thyroid replacement. At about the same time, she developed bronchitis; a chest X-ray and a CAT scan revealed pneumonia and enlarged lymph nodes. A biopsy confirmed that she had sarcoidosis, a disease that produces microscopic clumps of inflammatory cells in different parts of the body. But a six-month regimen of steroids resolved her symptoms.

Georgia was thirty pounds overweight and had slightly elevated blood pressure. Some of her teeth were crowned, and one was missing. Her skin was tender to the touch, especially around her neck, shoulders, lower back, and hips. Her shins hurt when pressure was applied, and she had an enlarged right knee. She had an abnormal blood test due to her thyroid disease.

What's important about Georgia's problems was that three culprits—dietary imbalance, vitamin D deficiency, and poorly toned muscles—were the common denominators that tied all of the symptoms and the diseases together.

Georgia got much better simply by taking adequate vitamin D and magnesium supplementation, making better food choices, and becoming more active.

In two months, she got much better on the Vitamin D Cure program, and you can, too. The upbeat message: you can not only stop disease, but you can actually reverse it!

Georgia's story isn't unusual at all; I see patients like her every day. Having taken care of adults and children with arthritis since 1995, I have had more than 55,000 patient encounters that have taught me that all of the symptoms and the diseases Georgia experienced are preventable.

Using Sunlight to Increase Your Vitamin D

Just as I told Georgia, one way to increase your vitamin D level is to increase your sun exposure, but this requires regular exposure to a UV index of 3 or greater. Most people need vitamin D supplementation to get the job done.

To estimate the amount of sun you need to make an adequate amount of vitamin D, follow these instructions from the Sun Exposure Times chart.

1. To estimate the amount of sun you need to make enough vitamin D, go to www.thevitamindcure.com and use the UV calculator. Enter your zip code and skin type, and you can calculate the minutes of sun exposure you need where you live.

2. Or you can go to http://www.epa.gov/enviro/facts/uv/uv_query .html and enter your zip code to calculate your UV index. This number isn't the real-time UV index—it's the estimated UV index at solar noon for a particular zip code. You can also download an app for your mobile device at: http://apps.usa.gov/uvindex/

3. Refer to the following chart to find your UVI (UV index) on the top row.

4. Follow this down and across to your skin type (see the definitions below the chart).

5. The number of minutes of exposure without sunscreen at least three times a week shown in the box gives you adequate vitamin D production to maintain a normal blood level. This is based on 50 to 75 percent skin exposure (shorts and T-shirt or swimsuit).

Note: Australia has a national program that provides real-time UV index values.

SUN EXPOSURE TIMES REQUIRED TO MAKE VITAMIN D

	UVI 0–2	UVI 3–5	UVI 6–7	UVI 8–10	UVI 11+
Type 1	No D	10–15	5–10	2–8	1–5
Type 2	No D	15–20	10–15	5–10	2–8
Type 3	No D	20–30	15–20	10–15	5–10
Type 4	No D	30–40	20–30	15–20	10–15
Types 5–6	No D	40–60	30–40	20–30	15–20

Double the exposure time if you are fifty or older.

A tanning bed is roughly equivalent to UVI 7–8.

Skin types

1   Always burn, never tan

2   Burn easily, rarely tan

3   Occasionally burn, slowly tan

4   Rarely burn, rapidly tan

5–6   Never burn, always dark

You should consider applying SPF 15 sunscreen or covering up after you have been exposed for the times listed in the chart. Although your body dissipates vitamin D slowly, if your winter (UV index below 3) is three months or longer, I recommend taking vitamin D supplements at least during the winter.

You can never make too much vitamin D from sun exposure because excess vitamin D is automatically inactivated in your skin by further sun exposure. So a person with a normal vitamin D level of 50 who spends a day on a boat with friends won't overdose on vitamin D. Most of the vitamin D made while on the boat will be inactivated by continued sun exposure. The UVB facilitation of vitamin D production is a self-regulating process.

Recent research suggests that people who frequent tanning salons have normal vitamin D levels, typically higher than 45. This would mean that if you're frequenting a tanning salon or you tan in your own tanning bed, you probably won't need vitamin D supplementation.

How Much Vitamin D Do You Need?

By this point in reading this book, you know that sun alone probably won't be your answer to vitamin D deficiency, mainly because no one spends enough time outdoors anymore. Furthermore, sun exposure may not be an option for some people—those who take certain medications or have certain medical conditions (e.g., lupus).

Also, we know that obese people aren't as efficient at making vitamin D from sunlight as people with normal weight. Those who are overweight may do better with supplements or a combination of supplements and sun rather than just sun exposure alone.

How do you figure out what kind of supplements you need and where you can get the right kind?

One Size Does Not Fit All

Vitamin D is fat-soluble. The bigger you are, the more D you need. When it comes to vitamin D supplements, one size doesn't fit all.

Drawing on information that Drs. Robert Heaney and Michael Holick published in the *American Journal of Clinical Nutrition*, I chose a weight-based calculation method to determine the amount of vitamin D you need. This takes body size into account when determining the appropriate replacement dose.

Here's how you should supplement vitamin D if you don't want to bother with measuring your vitamin D level. Just figure out your risk profile score and use that number to arrive at the right dose. Remember, too, that this may overestimate or underestimate your actual needs.

RISK SCORE AND DAILY DOSE OF VITAMIN D	
Risk Score	Daily Dose of D
0–2	No supplements; only sun (get blood level measured)
3–5	20 IU/lb. body weight
>5	25 IU/lb. body weight

Based on data from the Centers for Disease Control and Prevention (CDC), average vitamin D levels are 15 to 35. Because the ideal level is 40 to 60, this tells us that the average American probably needs 20 to 25 IU per pound of body weight to raise his or her vitamin D level to 40 to 60.

For good health, the minimum normal vitamin D level is 30. Toxicity—almost impossible to reach accidentally, by the way—would require a level of more than 250. In fact, if you have a vitamin D level of 60, you could still sunbathe or tan in a tanning bed and not experience toxicity. Similarly, if your level was 60 and you took 20 IU per pound, you would not become toxic. Your vitamin D level probably would approach 90, but unless you were taking excessive amounts of calcium, this would not result in toxicity. At the same time, it's important to remember that if you're tanning, you probably won't need supplementation.

Likewise, if you were a shut-in who never saw the light of day and your vitamin D level was 5, you could take 25 IU per pound and your vitamin D level would rise to 40. So even if you're not measuring your blood level, you can assume that doses of 20 to 25 IU per pound (or 40 to 60 IU per kilogram) daily based on your risk score will produce a vitamin D level in the normal range.

On the other hand, if you do choose to measure your vitamin D level via tests, you'll be able to adjust your vitamin D level by a specific amount (see the following chart for weight-based doses in units of vitamin D per pound). For example, if your vitamin D level at winter's end (March) is 15 and you want to tack on 35 more points to reach 50, you should take 26 units per pound to raise your vitamin D level about 35 points.

So if you weigh 170 pounds, you need 5,780 units of vitamin D a day. Round off your amount to 6,000 IU a day, and then check your vitamin D level in about three months. Remember, you may be getting additional D from daily vitamins or mineral supplements, and you need to include that in your calculated daily dose.

CALCULATING YOUR VITAMIN D DOSE FROM BLOOD LEVEL

Desired Change in Blood Level		Amount of Vitamin D_3 to Take	
ng/mL	nmol/L	IU/lb.	IU/kg.
5	12	4	9
10	25	8	17
15	37	11	24
20	50	15	34
25	62	19	42
30	75	23	51
35	87	26	60
40	100	30	67
45	112	34	76
50	125	38	84
55	137	41	93
60	150	45	101
65	162	49	109

The two forms of vitamin D are

1. Vitamin D_2 (ergocalciferol or Drisdol, the prescription form of D_2)

2. Vitamin D_3 (cholecalciferol, which is not prescribed in the United States, but is available over the counter)

D_2 comes from plants. Mammals make D_3 from cholesterol with the assistance of UVB radiation and heat.

In about seven days, a human's vitamin D_2 dose is half-metabolized; complete elimination takes two weeks. A dose of vitamin D_3 is metabolized in half in about ten weeks. Peak blood levels of vitamin D_2 are 30 percent lower than D_3 after the same dose.

You must take doses of vitamin D_2 at least twice a week and preferably daily to adjust for rapid elimination and lower peak levels. In general, a weekly or monthly dose of 50,000 IU D_2 won't produce an adequate rise in vitamin D levels or vitamin D effects. A recent review on the effects of vitamin D on bone confirms the inefficacy of vitamin D_2 as it is commonly prescribed.

Vitamin D_3 replacement at a given dose will reach steady state in ten weeks. The long half-life of vitamin D_3 allows for missed doses without a significant drop in blood level. Makeup doses and weekly or monthly dosing are acceptable and will still maintain a steady blood level.

You can buy vitamin D_3 over the counter at a low cost—a year's supply of gel caps for less than $20. The co-pay for prescription vitamin D_2 may cost about as much as you would pay for a year's supply of over-the-counter D_3. For all these reasons, I suggest you skip the prescription D_2.

You can take your vitamin D_3 once a week or only on certain days, as long as your weekly total is based on your needs. For example, if you need 3,000 IU a day, you can take 21,000 IU once a week or 4,000 IU five days a week for a total of 20,000 IU. The difference of 1,000 IU for the week is negligible. For any extended period of time, you shouldn't need any more than 40 units per pound or 85 units per kilogram. Even if you're living in a submarine, this dose raises your blood level by 50 points.

This table also works in reverse, so you can use it to adjust your dose down if your vitamin D level is too high after taking supplements. Just reduce your intake by the specified amount. When reducing your dose, these data can overcorrect. An alternate method of reducing your D level is to drop your dose by 25 percent (daily or weekly total) and check your level again in two months.

Remember that brief sun exposure can spike your vitamin D level temporarily, so don't measure your levels following inconsistent sun exposure—such as on the day you return from a trip to Hawaii.

Suppose you find out that your vitamin D level is 95 after your initial calculations because you didn't take into account the vitamin D you were getting via the sun or other supplements. To reduce your level by 40 ($95 - 40 = 55$), simply decrease your intake by 30 IU per pound and measure your level again in three months. If this method overcorrects your vitamin D level, then the elevated level may have been related to recent sun exposure, or your initial calculation overestimated your needs.

Let's say the 95 was your measurement after you'd been taking 25 IU per pound for three months without previously measuring your blood level. This means you probably had a normal vitamin D level to begin with, so maybe you don't need supplementation.

Vitamin D requirements may be different after fat stores are saturated, which alters the characteristics of vitamin D metabolism in extreme obesity if your body mass index is higher than 35. Very few studies have examined vitamin D metabolism in the morbidly obese, but it does appear that compared to those who are not obese, overweight folks have a diminished response to UVB production of vitamin D.

If you weigh 300 pounds or more, the above calculations may slightly overestimate or underestimate your needs. Rounding down dose calculations and monitoring your D level every two months will provide the information you need to adjust your dosing safely.

Vitamin D Is Critical for Kids

Children, especially during infancy and in preschool years, are at greater risk for vitamin D deficiency than many adults. A study in Pittsburgh revealed that 92 percent of African American newborns and 66 percent of European American newborns had vitamin D levels less than 30 nanograms per milliliter. And the infants had lower vitamin D levels than their mothers. This also means that they had vitamin D deficiency during development in the uterus.

You can use the same formulas and tables for children and infants. According to my observations and those of Dr. Armin Zittermann, weight-based dosing is the same for children as for adults. We know that it is absolutely critical to have normal vitamin D levels during pregnancy and early childhood to prevent infections, osteoporosis, autoimmune diseases, and cancer. If this is the only message you embrace from *The Vitamin D Cure*, you will have changed the health of your family for generations to come.

JENNIFER'S LEG PAIN AND POOR SLEEP

Jennifer was four when her parents first brought her to the Arthritis Institute; her family doctor wanted us to investigate the severe pain in her legs, especially the right knee. She'd complained of pain for about eight months, and her physician was concerned that she might have juvenile arthritis.

The problem sometimes interfered with her daily activities, but rubbing helped relieve the pain, which she experienced at night. She had an elevated antinuclear antibody test.

We knew that she was a full-term baby who was breast-fed for two years (the first year Jennifer had no vitamin or formula supplementation at all).

I saw no swollen joints or rashes that would point to juvenile arthritis. Her shins were tender to pressure. Her general health was normal. Her lab tests revealed a vitamin D level of 24, with a normal calcium and PTH.

I put her on vitamin D at 1,142 IU per day or 30 IU per pound per day in a liquid preparation that was 2,000 IU per drop. We instructed Mom to give Jennifer 4 drops on Sunday, or 8,000 IU per week. I also encouraged Jennifer's mother to feed her more fresh vegetables, fruits, and lean protein and to avoid salt, cheese, and grains.

I knew that the amount we had prescribed wasn't toxic, because thirty years ago, public health policy in the Netherlands had mandated that all newborns receive 2,000 IU of vitamin D (in cod liver oil) to prevent rickets, and there were no observations of any toxicity.

How did Jennifer do? Her first-visit scores and notes looked like this:

- 0.375–65–0–15–6 (function, pain, fatigue, health perception, sleep)
- 90 minutes of stiffness in the morning

At follow-up four months later, though, the changes looked like this:

- 0.125–0–15–5–6 scores
- No stiffness
- Function improved by 67 percent
- Pain completely resolved
- 67 percent improvement in her overall perceived health
- Vitamin D level of 41

At a later follow-up visit, Jennifer's mother said she had run out of the vitamin D liquid, and her daughter's leg pains had returned in several weeks. After that, she resumed the supplementation and diet improvements, which relieved the symptoms.

Jennifer's experiences highlight the vulnerability of children to vitamin D and dietary deficiencies. Aches and pains in kids aren't always just growing pains, as many people think.

This also underscores one risk of breast-feeding. Breast milk has little or no vitamin D unless the mother's vitamin D level is 45 to 60. This is why all women who breast-feed should supplement their breast-fed infant, or take enough vitamin D to normalize their own vitamin D level. Dr. Bruce Hollis of the Medical University of South Carolina found that the average nursing mother required 4,000 IU or more of vitamin D a day to optimize vitamin D concentrations in breast milk and normalize blood levels in the infants. He is currently studying the safe upper limits of vitamin D supplementation during pregnancy.

The American Academy of Pediatrics recommends 200 IU of vitamin D a day for an infant up to two months of age who doesn't take supplemental formula. This ruling takes it for granted that a breast-feeding mother is probably vitamin D deficient and that her breast milk has no vitamin D.

If you assume that an average newborn infant weighs about eight pounds, giving a baby 20 to 25 IU per pound will amount to 160 to 200 IU of vitamin D a day, which is exactly what the American Academy of Pediatrics recommends. In my experience, it's hard to get children to take vitamin D supplements, but parents can give liquid vitamin D instead of capsules.

Tips on Buying Vitamin D Supplements

When The *Vitamin D Cure* was first published, vitamin D supplements were hard to find, especially in doses greater than 400 IU. Since that time, though, numerous companies have begun to manufacture and distribute vitamin D.

Here are some handy guidelines on buying supplements:

- Buy vitamin D_3, not D_2. This is the vitamin D your body makes from sunlight. It hangs around longer in your blood, which allows for once-a-week dosing, unlike vitamin D_2, which must be dosed daily to be close in efficacy. Most over-the-counter vitamin D sold in the United States is vitamin D_3. This is not the case in Europe. (See page 206 in the Q&A Appendix for more information.)

- Stick to major distributors of vitamin D. You can choose from a number of reliable brands. Generally speaking, the larger the company distributing the product, the higher the quality and the lower the price. A few companies that make high-quality, low-cost vitamin D are Carlson Labs, Now Foods, Swanson Health Products, Jarrow Formulas, Nature Made, and Solgar. You can also buy national store-brand vitamin D of reliable quality at Wal-Mart, Costco, CVS, and Walgreens.

- In liquid vitamin D, buy Ddrops of Canada (www.ddrops.ca). This is the only liquid vitamin D with a patented precise gravity-fed dropper top. You invert the bottle, and it delivers exactly the same size drop of liquid every time. Manual droppers and squeeze bottles, in contrast, deliver drops of different sizes, which make accurate dosing difficult. This can be problematic when you are supplementing the vitamin D of infants and children.

• Don't pay more than $20 for a year's supply of vitamin D. This figure will vary according to the size dose you take, of course. Keep in mind that the price of vitamin D supplements has dropped by more than half since 2008. Paying more doesn't give you higher-quality supplements.

Most people have better tolerance for vitamin D gel caps and drops than for tablets combined with calcium. The majority of vitamin D tablets are combined with calcium, even though the label may not indicate that this is the case. The problem is that calcium tends to cause constipation and stomach upset in some people. Tablets with calcium would be especially troublesome if you're dosing with vitamin D weekly.

Stay Away from Too Much Vitamin A

When you're shopping for vitamin D, avoid supplements with vitamin A in them. If you do take vitamin D supplements that contain vitamin A, be careful because you can easily overdose on A when you're innocently trying to beef up your D level. Worse yet, too much vitamin A can negate the benefits of vitamin D.

The combination D/A products are derived from fish liver oil (usually cod-liver oil), and the typical ratio is 10:1, meaning 10 times more vitamin A than vitamin D. The new RDI/DRI for vitamin A is 2,310 IU for women, 3,000 IU for men, and about half that for children. So you get a toxic amount at about 9,000 to 10,000 IU per day in adults and 3,000 IU per day in children. A better, safer form of vitamin A is beta-carotene.

You can recognize acute vitamin A intoxication by the following symptoms:

• Nausea   • Blurred vision

• Vomiting   • Rashes

- Headaches
- Lack of coordination
- Dizziness

Keep in mind, too, that chronic vitamin A toxicity can cause birth defects, liver abnormalities, osteoporosis, and central nervous system disorders, so this isn't a vitamin you can take lightly.

Many people worry about taking too much vitamin D, but it's very hard to overdose on vitamin D. Toxicity is highly unlikely at a vitamin D level of less than 250 ng/mL and at a vitamin D intake of less than 60 IU per pound, or 10,000 IU a day.

You can spot toxic vitamin D levels by the following symptoms:

- Frequent urination
- Constipation
- Nausea
- Weakness
- Vomiting
- Weight loss
- Poor appetite

You may also have increased blood levels of calcium, which results in increased urination, dehydration, lethargy, and confusion. Chronic elevations of blood calcium can cause deposits of calcium and phosphate in your skin, muscles, and internal organs, such as the kidneys.

Ideal or high vitamin D levels, combined with too much calcium supplementation, will increase your risk of kidney stone formation, especially if you don't adopt the Vitamin D Cure diet. If you're supplementing vitamin D, be careful, because you probably don't need calcium supplements (see chapter 7).

If you think you've taken too much vitamin D or vitamin A, call your physician immediately. You need to have your blood levels checked. Then your doctor can use those results to decide on appropriate treatment.

6

Step Three: Reduce Your Acid Excess by Changing Your Diet

A key part of the Vitamin D Cure is Step Three: the defining moment when you calculate your acid excess and rebalance your diet. You start by figuring out what your acid excess is. You identify your dietary weaknesses. Then you eliminate salt, cheese, pasta, cereal, and bread.

Check out the amounts of produce and lean protein you eat daily. Set your sights on consuming *at least* half a gram of protein per pound of lean body weight a day. As a basic rule, eat three times as much produce as lean protein.

Survey What You Eat

Before you fill out your dietary survey, read the following information on the nine food categories. This will help you complete the survey more accurately.

1. Cereal: This includes cereals made from grains, such as wheat, barley, oats, rice, corn, quinoa, and any other grain that's old or new, whole or processed. In other words, all cereals!

2. Bread: This means white, wheat, oat, whole, multigrain, or otherwise. If it's bread, it counts.

3. Pasta: All pasta counts, regardless of composition—seminole wheat, whole grain, flax, egg noodles, rice noodles, and spinach.

4. Meat/Fish: This includes beef, pork, poultry, game meat, organ meat, and seafood of any kind (including shellfish). I also include cottage cheese. Don't forget processed meat—bacon, sausage, smoked meats, cured meats, most lunch meats, and commercial jerky. Processed meats contain lots of salt, so answer yes to the salt question if you eat processed meats.

5. Beans: These are legumes. This category includes kidney beans, navy beans, chili beans, garbanzo beans, peas, lima beans, soybeans, and peanuts.

6. Nuts: This group includes, for example, walnuts, almonds, cashews, pecans, pistachios, macadamia nuts, and Brazil nuts.

7. Cheese: Here I'm referring to hard and soft cheeses of all kinds except cottage cheese, which falls into the meat category. Cottage cheese is lower in acid but provides only about half as much protein as lean meat per equivalent serving.

8. Fruits: The fruit group includes all kinds of whole fruits, along with canned fruits and fruit juices. That means 100 percent fruit juices only; fruit-flavored drinks are not fruit juice.

9. Vegetables: The veggie group encompasses all kinds of fresh or frozen vegetables. If you regularly eat canned vegetables, including canned tomatoes, you must answer "yes" to the following question regarding salt because of the salt they contain.

Check a box on the following worksheet for every serving you consumed in the past twenty-four hours.

DIETARY ACID-BASE WORKSHEET

Acid Foods

Cereal	☐ ☐ ☐ ☐ ☐ ☐	Total _____ × 8 = _____
Bread	☐ ☐ ☐ ☐ ☐ ☐	Total _____ × 2 = _____
Pasta	☐ ☐ ☐ ☐ ☐ ☐	Total _____ × 6 = _____
Meat/fish	☐ ☐ ☐ ☐ ☐ ☐	Total _____ × 9 = _____
Beans	☐ ☐ ☐ ☐ ☐ ☐	Total _____ × 4 = _____
Nuts	☐ ☐ ☐ ☐ ☐ ☐	Total _____ × 7 = _____
Cheese	☐ ☐ ☐ ☐ ☐ ☐	Total _____ × 20 = _____

Acid Foods Total _____

Alkaline Foods

Fruits	☐ ☐ ☐ ☐ ☐ ☐	Total _____ × 3 = _____
Vegetables	☐ ☐ ☐ ☐ ☐ ☐	Total _____ × 3 = _____

Alkaline Foods Total _____

Do you add salt, cook with salt, or eat salty foods
at more than three meals a week?   ☐ Yes   ☐ No

Regarding saturated fat, do you eat butter,
shortening, cream, ice cream, and/or
processed meats at more than three
meals a week?   ☐ Yes   ☐ No

Scoring the Survey

1. Add your total number of servings in each row, and multiply by the factor on the right to come up with a total score for each food category.

2. Now go down the right side of the survey and add up the Acid Foods Total and the Alkaline Foods Total.

3. If you answered "yes" to the question on salt or to the question on saturated fat, subtract 3 points from your Alkaline Foods Total for each "yes" answer, or add 3 points to your Acid Foods Total for each if your Alkaline Foods Total is already 0.

4. Now subtract your Alkaline Foods Total from your Acid Foods Total.

5. This is your acid excess.

Acid Foods Total – Alkaline Foods Total = Acid Excess

Interpreting Your Acid Excess Score

<0   Good for you! You have your acid excess well in tow. No worries.

0–10   Minimal problem with acid excess. Has an easy fix.

11–20 Moderate acid excess. Requires some tweaking.

21–30 High acid excess. Really needs a fixer-upper!

>30   Very high acid excess. You need help!

Don't feel bad if your score isn't acceptable. Most people have acid excess. Most of my patients post acid excess figures that are 30 or higher, and before I changed my diet, mine was 20. All you have to do is just use this information to make meaningful changes to your diet.

Acid excess simply means you're not getting enough potassium and magnesium in the form of fruits and vegetables, you're consuming far too many acid-producing foods, or both.

Make some moves to fix this problem because it's important to stop what's pulling potassium, magnesium, and calcium from your muscles and bones, to balance your body chemistry.

If you're deficient in both vitamin D and magnesium and unable to absorb an adequate amount of calcium from your diet, you'll zap even more calcium from your bones. Don't sacrifice the health of your muscles and bones, or everything attached to your skeleton will start coming apart.

The Balancing Act

Acid excess isn't really very complicated. Four things people commonly eat that lead to acid excess are:

1. Salt

2. Cheese and saturated fat

3. Too many servings of grain-based foods

4. Too few green vegetables and fruits

Studying your answers to the food survey will spotlight your own problem areas. Consider the following example of a typical American eating pattern, and you can see how the dietary flaws cause trouble.

In this typical American menu, acid reigns.

DIETARY ACID-BASE EXAMPLE: THE TYPICAL AMERICAN DIET

Acid Foods

Cereal	☒ ☐ ☐ ☐ ☐ ☐	Total	1 × 8 =	8
Bread	☒ ☒ ☒ ☐ ☐ ☐	Total	3 × 2 =	6
Pasta	☒ ☐ ☐ ☐ ☐ ☐	Total	1 × 7 =	7
Meat/Fish	☒ ☒ ☐ ☐ ☐ ☐	Total	2 × 9 =	18
Beans	☐ ☐ ☐ ☐ ☐ ☐	Total	___ × 4 = ___	
Nuts	☐ ☐ ☐ ☐ ☐ ☐	Total	___ × 7 = ___	
Cheese	☒ ☐ ☐ ☐ ☐ ☐	Total	1 × 20 =	20

Acid Foods Total 59

Alkaline Foods

Fruits	☒ ☐ ☐ ☐ ☐ ☐	Total	1 × 3 = 3
Vegetables	☒ ☐ ☐ ☐ ☐ ☐	Total	1 × 3 = 3

Alkaline Foods Total 6

Do you add salt, cook with salt, or eat salty foods at more than three meals a week?

Yes, so I subtract 3 from my Alkaline Foods Total, leaving 3.

Regarding saturated fat, do you eat butter, shortening, cream, ice cream, and/or processed meats at more than three meals a week?

Yes, so I subtract another 3 points from my Alkaline Foods Total, leaving 0.

59 – 0 = Acid Excess of 59

In the example above, here's what this individual ate during a single day:

• Breakfast: cereal and toast with coffee

- Lunch: sandwich (two slices of bread, lunch meat, cheese) and a diet drink
- Dinner: lasagna (meat, cheese, pasta), salad, and bread with a diet drink

This is a bad diet for sure, with cereal, pasta, and bread generating 21 points of acid. That's more than a third of the acid excess. Another 20 points of acid come from cheese alone. So this person got 41 points of acid from foods that provide very little nutrition. And the small amount of good nutrition in those foods automatically gets nullified by the acid they produce and the bad fat they contain. Saturated fat reduces your kidneys' ability to dump acid; the salt leads to urinating extra potassium, magnesium, and calcium.

If you're still dead set on the idea of eating lots of salt, cheese, pasta, cereal, and bread, keep in mind that for good health, you'll have to increase your fruit and vegetable intake by twenty servings! You'd better be hungry because you'll need a cow-size stomach to take in that much food.

Obviously, you can't do it, so the only option is cutting out the acid. The only practical solution is to eliminate low-nutrition foods that produce acid and/or contain bad fats. Also, start eating lean meat instead of processed meats. This means no prepared, preserved meats. That will get you down to an Acid Foods Total of 18. The equation looks like this:

$$18 - 6 = \text{Acid Excess of } 12$$

You can easily balance your body chemistry by increasing your produce intake by four more servings. This will give you a total of six servings, and your acid excess drops to 0.

So you say, "Hey, you just removed half of my food, so now I'm starving." That may be your knee-jerk reaction, but the fact is, you now have room to eat another healthy meal. In addition, nutrient-dense food satisfies you with fewer calories.

Eat the Right Stuff

"What *can* I eat?" That will probably be your first question after you finish taking your food inventory. But the answer is really simple, because eating the right stuff just means sticking to two food groups: lean meat and fresh produce. That's easy to remember and easy to do. The two simple rules are:

1. Eat mostly from two food groups: lean meat and fresh produce.
2. Consume three times as much fresh produce as lean meat by weight (3:1 produce to protein).

By lean protein, we mean lean animal protein. This includes grass-fed beef; pork tenderloin; seafood (all kinds, but especially those high in omega-3 fat); boneless, skinless poultry; game meat; and, to a lesser extent, omega eggs (these are eggs labeled "higher in omega-3" because the hens get better feed).

The word "lean" means meat with little or no saturated fat, and the animals the meat comes from should be fed grass (grass and clover)—not grain! If you're looking for organic meats, watch for terms such as "pasture-fed," "grass-fed," and "clover-fed" animals. When shopping for organic meats, read the label information that specifies the composition of the feed used. But always remember that even more important than trying to find organic meat is eating a greater amount of lean meat.

The problem is, when cattle handlers fatten their cattle for slaughter, they send them to the feedlot and give them an unlimited mixture of corn and soybeans, which marbles their meat and liver with saturated fats and increases their body mass, just as it does in humans. Conversely, a grass-fed cow is a lean cow whose meat is higher in omega-3 fats, monounsaturated fats, and polyunsaturated fats. These fats improve your kidneys' ability to excrete acid, lower your blood pressure, lower your triglycerides, and raise your good cholesterol. They also decrease production of inflammatory substances that accelerate damage to your blood vessels and lead to heart attacks and strokes and that aggravate inflammatory diseases such as rheumatoid arthritis.

The amount of protein you eat determines how much produce you need to eat. The American Dietetic Association lists protein requirements at 0.8 gram per kilogram of body weight, or 0.36 gram per pound of body weight. Research reviewed by Dr. Peter Lemon of the University of

Western Ontario in the *Journal of the American College of Nutrition* suggests that people who are physically active may require 1.6 grams per kilogram, or about twice as much protein a day to meet metabolic needs than was previously thought. After studying bone metabolism in elderly women, Dr. Jane Kerstetter of the University of Connecticut says in the *American Journal of Clinical Nutrition* that healthy women need an average of 1.2 grams per kilogram per day, or 0.55 gram per pound of body weight of protein per day to maintain bone mass. New research suggests that children may have daily protein requirements as high as 0.7 to 0.8 gram per pound of lean body weight.

Your protein intake should be about half your ideal body weight in grams. A 150-pound person needs a protein intake of 75 grams per day.

Using the following chart, you can figure out how much meat you need to eat to get enough daily protein.

MINIMUM DAILY PROTEIN REQUIREMENT

Minimum Daily Protein Requirement by Ideal Body Weight*

Height (in)	IBW (lbs)	IBW (kg)	Protein (g)
58	105	48	58
59	109	50	60
60	112	51	62
61	116	53	64
62	120	55	66
63	124	56	68
64	128	58	70
65	132	60	73
66	136	62	75
67	140	64	77
68	144	65	79
69	149	68	82
70	153	70	84
71	157	71	86
72	162	74	89
73	166	75	91
74	171	78	94
75	176	80	97
76	180	82	99

*Ideal body weight is defined as your weight if you had a body mass index of 22.

Fresh produce refers to uncooked, unfrozen, and unprocessed vegetables and fruits. Canned vegetables are often blanched in boiling water before canning, and manufacturers add salt to increase shelf life. Most manufacturers of canned fruits add sugar for preservation. Frozen produce is sometimes blanched before freezing, and a significant number of nutrients are lost in the blanching process.

Think of it like this:

- Fresh is best.

- Frozen is okay when you're in a bind. (Choose fresh-frozen.)

- Canned is okay if you're stranded on a desert island.

If you do use canned produce or meat, rinse it to get rid of the added salt and sugar.

The produce-to-protein ratio of 3:1 comes from acid-base calculations that were adapted from Drs. Thomas Remer and Friedrich Manz at the Research Institute of Child Nutrition in Dortmund, Germany. A 3.5-ounce serving of lean meat produces about 9 points of acid. The average 3.5-ounce serving of fruit or vegetable produces about 3 points of antacid. That means that if you want to neutralize the acid from one serving of lean meat, you must eat three servings of fresh produce.

This 3:1 ratio, in conjunction with the elimination of salt, can help to reverse the modern inversion of the potassium-to-sodium ratio, which Drs. Anthony Sebastian and Lynda Frassetto at the University of California, San Francisco, link to high blood pressure, kidney stones, and osteoporosis. How much produce does a 150-pound person need? Three ounces of lean meat give you about 25 grams of protein, so your protein requirement is 75 grams, or 9 ounces of lean meat per day. To meet the ratio of 3:1 produce to protein, you should eat 3 × 9 or 27 ounces of produce each day.

Breakfast Management

I had trouble switching from my ritualistic breakfast bowl of steel-cut oats, oat bran, walnuts, and raisins. The first week or two felt strange, and I often caught myself reaching for the bowl and the gallon of milk.

I can tell you that Mr. McCormick, Mr. Kellogg, Mr. Pillsbury, and the other grain titans have been excellent marketers, and this is one reason they have traditionally owned breakfast.

People tend to balk when they find out that they're not really supposed to have toast, cereal, bagels, doughnuts, pancakes, or waffles. And when they have to digest the idea of a lean pork chop for breakfast, this may not be an easy transition.

But look at the convenience aspect—it's really easy to reheat leftovers from your dinner last night.

Here are some examples of healthy breakfasts that won't leave you hungry a few hours later. (By the way, making this breakfast change eliminated my post-oatmeal heartburn.)

Option 1

3 eggs minus 2 yolks to cut the fat (boiled, poached, or scrambled)

2 cups fresh spinach leaves

1 medium-sized tomato, sliced

½ avocado

Universal Marinade (homemade earlier in the week)

1 banana

2 glasses of water

Preparation time: < 5 minutes

Don't worry about calories. Eat all you want of this healthy stuff. Quick tip: boil a dozen eggs at a time and refrigerate them so you have handy options available.

Option 2

4 ounces grilled pork tenderloin (grilled over the weekend)

1 cup steamed asparagus (from last night's dinner)

1 cup small red potatoes, boiled and then sautéed in olive oil with garlic (from dinner)

1 whole sliced orange

4 ounces hot green tea

Preparation time: < 5 minutes

Calories: It's all healthy. Eat all you want!

Lunch to Go

Most people want a lunch that's quick and easy. Many of us have to grab lunch on the run, so we have no prep time. Here are some things you can do that work *for* your health:

- Refrigerate a container of chopped walnuts and flax meal. It goes great with fresh fruit. This is a convenient source of protein and healthy fats that requires no preparation. (And most offices have a refrigerator.)
- Eat leftovers from dinner for lunch.
- Avoid junk food. And if you do want to snack on something you can't resist, just be sure to fill yourself up by eating your healthy foods first. Then you can use your remaining appetite for chocolate-covered nuts or raisins.
- Keep fresh fruit handy for you, your coworkers, and your family. This simple move will make people around you eat less trash food.

Option 1
½ cup chopped walnuts with flax meal
1 banana dipped in walnut mix
1 apple

Option 2
1 boiled egg
1 banana dipped in walnuts and flax meal
1 orange

Doing Dinner Right

What if your spouse, kids, or partner refuses to eat this way? Then you just cook your own meals; that's what I've done since I switched to this diet. Believe me, not everyone wants to eat this healthy. Many people say, "Hey, I don't feel really bad, so why change?"

But since you're the one doing the health upgrade, schedule some weekend time to cook a large amount of lean meat. Make enough boneless, skinless chicken, pork tenderloin, or seafood for two people, two meals a day—or about ten meals. That's usually enough for a busy working couple. Steam or sauté about three days' worth of vegetables. Also, make available (at home and work) large cases of fresh fruit.

For dinner you can have lean meats, and Universal Marinade (see the recipes) can double as a salad dressing and a seasoning for vegetables. See www.eatwild.com for farms that produce organic produce and grass-fed animal meat.

Lean Meats

Seafood (wild-caught instead of farmed; canned in a pinch; always drain and rinse)

Salmon	Perch
Halibut	Catfish
Tuna	Shrimp
Trout	Scallops
Bass	Lobster
Walleye	Crab

Lean beef (preferably grass-fed and trimmed of all fat)

Flank steak

Top sirloin

London broil

Beef tenderloin

Ground eye of round (5 percent fat or less; drain fat after cooking)

Lean pork

Pork tenderloin

Butterfly pork chops from loin

Boneless skinless poultry

Chicken breast	Emu
Turkey breast	Pheasant
Ostrich (fresh)	Quail
Wild turkey	

Omega eggs

Omega eggs are labeled "higher in omega-3" because the hens get better feed.

Game meat

Rabbit	Caribou
Venison	Elk

NUTRITIONAL COMPOSITION OF LEAN PROTEINS

Food	Preparation	Serving (g.) (oz.)	Protein (g.)	Fat (g.)	CHO (g.)	Calories
Chicken, boneless, skinless breast	Roasted	86 (½ breast)	26.7	3.0	0	142
Turkey, boneless, skinless breast	Roasted	87 (3 oz.)	26.2	0.6	0	117
Pork tenderloin trimmed of fat	Broiled	85 (3 oz.)	25.9	5.4	0	159
Salmon, Atlantic, wild-caught	Baked	85 (3 oz.)	21.6	6.9	0	155
Salmon, Atlantic, farmed	Baked	85 (3 oz.)	18.8	10.5	0	175
Salmon, coho, wild-caught	Baked	85 (3 oz.)	19.9	3.7	0	118
Salmon, coho, farmed	Baked	85 (3 oz.)	20.7	7.0	0	151
Tuna, blue fin	Baked	85 (3 oz.)	25.4	5.3	0	156
Tuna, canned	Canned	85 (3 oz.)	21.7	0.7	0	99
Shrimp, mixed variety, in the shell	Boiled	85 (3 oz.)	17.8	0.9	0	84
Venison, 1-inch loin steak	Broiled	85 (3 oz.)	25.7	2.0	0	128
Venison tenderloin	Broiled	85 (3 oz.)	25.4	2.0	0	127
Egg, chicken	Boiled	1 egg	6.0	5.0	0.6	78

Cutting Salt

Recent research shows that high salt (sodium chloride) intake causes your kidneys to break down and discard vitamin D. In essence, salt creates a leak in your vitamin D bucket. Baked chicken and grilled meat minus salt can be tough to swallow. The healthy alternative I use is fruit juice mixed with healthy oils. Citrus juices are natural meat tenderizers. Anyone who makes homemade barbecue sauce knows that pineapple juice is a staple ingredient. Lemon juice, commonly used to make fish more palatable, also is a natural meat tenderizer.

Try the following seasoning that's perfect for meats, vegetables, and salads. It will make you forget you ever thought you needed salt.

Universal Marinade/Dressing
   1 part freshly squeezed lemon juice
   2 parts oil (canola or olive or flaxseed)
   2 to 5 cloves garlic from a hand press
   1 teaspoon grated ginger, cumin, or curry (amount and spice choice to taste)
   Pepper to taste

Use any combination of fruit juices or puréed tomatoes to change the flavor. There's no salt, and the dressing gets its sourness and zing from the lemon or lime juice. Alternatively, use a vinegar, but make sure there's no salt added. If you want a little spice, add chili pepper or some grated jalapeño pepper.

Because citrus is a great natural meat tenderizer, you can use this to marinate your meats and vegetables when cooking. Fix jars of different flavors of marinades, and store in the refrigerator. Get your kids involved so they're on the bandwagon of better eating. Do lots of experimentation with your food so you can discover new ways to eat good foods that suit your palate.

Sampling Vegetables

Many of us didn't like vegetables when we were kids, and we still don't. As kids, we may have eaten tasteless stuff—canned or frozen spinach boiled in a pot, or frozen carrots and peas, or frozen bitter Brussels sprouts.

But now, mix it up a bit. Ever use fresh baby spinach leaves as a salad base or a pasta replacement? Spinach is an excellent source of magnesium and makes four times more antacid than most other vegetables per equivalent weighted serving. Or try fresh Brussels sprouts trimmed from the stalk, steamed, and then sautéed in olive oil and garlic.

Vegetables with lots of calcium

Bok choy

Kale

Broccoli

Chinese cabbage

Chinese mustard greens

Vegetables with lots of magnesium

Spinach (fresh leaf or baby leaf)

Potatoes (leave skins on)

Collard greens

Other vegetables loaded with nutrition

Artichokes

Asparagus

Peppers (green, red, orange, yellow)

Carrots

Garlic

Mushrooms of all kinds (sun-dried are rich in vitamin D)

Mustard greens

Onions

Parsley

Seaweed (kelp)

Swiss chard

Tomatoes

Greening Up and Graining Down

Italian Americans use pasta as the base for meat, vegetables, and cheese. Chinese Americans use noodles and rice, European Americans use bread, and Latin Americans use corn. These are all grains, which provide lots of carbohydrates, very little fiber, very little protein, and otherwise no nutrition. They actually work against you by increasing your acid load tremendously. Follow the motto "Choose green over grain."

The green base has more fiber, minerals (magnesium, potassium, calcium), antioxidants, vitamins (folic acid, vitamin C, vitamin K), and a whole host of nutrients. All of this comes in a package that has almost no calories and generates antacid to alkalinize your metabolism.

You can serve all of the meat entrées and the egg dishes on a bed of greens. Let the juices and the flavors from the meat and the vegetables serve as dressing, rather than separating the greens into a salad bowl. The interaction of textures and flavors makes the food interesting and tasty.

> 2 to 3 cups mixed greens or baby spinach leaves, washed and spun dry (or take kale, collard greens, or another large-leafed green vegetable and slice into ½- to 1-inch-wide strips and mix with other greens or serve alone)
> 1 large or 2 small tomatoes, sliced (or a handful of cherry tomatoes)
> ½ avocado, sliced
> ¼ cup dried cherries or fresh berries (blueberries, raspberries, strawberries, blackberries)
> 1 tablespoon Universal Marinade

Put the ingredients on a plate, and top with a serving of a meat or egg entrée of your choice (see the recipes in this book).

How about Nuts and Seeds?

Nuts are excellent sources of nutrition. Nutrient-dense, they make a great substitute for cheese in the North American diet and create only about a third of the acid that cheese does. Unlike cheese, though, they contain almost no salt (unless salt has been added), and they have mostly monounsaturated fat and substantial amounts of fiber.

Ground nuts add texture, flavor, and nutrition to salads, meat, and vegetables. Nuts are some of the richest sources of dietary magnesium.

Large studies of cardiovascular risk factors (weight and cholesterol) never show that nuts make you fatter or raise your cholesterol. In fact, people who consume nuts regularly usually have lower weight, lower cholesterol, and lower incidences of heart disease and diabetes. Recent studies show that nuts do not aggravate diverticulitis but actually may prevent this disease.

Here are some tips:

- Buy nuts in the shell or dry roasted without salt.
- Avoid nuts roasted in trans fat.
- Keep nuts in a dry, cool, dark place, or place them in a container in the refrigerator so oils in them won't turn rancid.
- Keep mixtures of different chopped nuts in the refrigerator to use in cooking.
- Remember that nuts are high in calories and omega-6 fats, so be careful not to overconsume.
- Eat plenty of the "best nuts" (walnuts and macadamia nuts have a very low omega-6 to omega-3 ratio: 4–6:1. An ideal ratio is 1–4:1).
- Hazelnuts produce net antacid after digestion.
- Flaxseed is loaded with alpha linolenic acid, an omega-3 fatty acid. (I use ground flaxseed sprinkled with chopped nuts to balance the omega-6 to omega-3 ratio.)
- Remember that peanuts are legumes, not nuts.

Here are two weeks of suggested menus. Experiment with your own—and enjoy!

Culinary talent requires curiosity, a hunger for experimentation, experience, passion, and no fear of failure. Our recipe creator, Chef Kelly, has been cooking since childhood and embodies all of these traits. She devours recipes from various sources. Then she modifies, mixes, and matches them to the specific requirements of the Vitamin D Cure. As practicality and budgets dictate, she can take leftover ingredients, study them, and prepare a tasty meal without anything going to waste. What follows are some examples of her magic. To learn more about Chef Kelly, go to www.tastesmilerepeat.com.

- Do your best to have two glasses of water with each meal. Switch it up by adding fruit wedges, fresh mint leaves, or cucumber slices.
- Be creative and have a little fun with your food.
- When cooking meat or vegetables, make a little extra for a meal the next day.
- Incorporate flavor and nutrients by adding your favorite herbs to olive oil or white wine vinegar to infuse the flavor; use this the same way you would use regular oil and vinegar.
- For a "creamy" variation without the guilt, puree an avocado with your favorite vinaigrette or the Universal Marinade, and top your meats, vegetables, and greens with this scrumptious concoction.
- Eat only when you are hungry, not out of habit. Snacks are optional.
- Always cook with olive oil, and use canola, flax, and walnut oil for dressings and other condiments that do not require high heat.

Vitamin D Cure Two-Week Meal Plan

Starred items (*) are included in the recipes section or elsewhere in the book.

Monday

Breakfast Avocado Scramble Wrap*
1 orange
Hot tea

Lunch Turkey breast with steamed asparagus, chopped tomatoes, sprouts, and Universal Marinade* in a romaine lettuce leaf
2 apricots

Snack 1 apple with 2 tablespoons Homemade Nut Butter*

Dinner Grilled chicken breast topped with Everyday Chimichurri*

Steamed broccoli and cauliflower

Tuesday

Breakfast Breakfast chicken salad. Combine one grilled chicken breast from the night before, 1 rib celery (chopped), a chopped apple, walnuts, and raisins, all mixed together with equal parts lemon juice and extra-virgin olive oil.

Seasonal fruit

Cup of coffee with ground cinnamon

Lunch Mixed greens with cucumbers, tomatoes, scallions, and Universal Marinade

Snack Kiwi with small handful of pistachios

Dinner Balsamic Marinated Skirt Steak with Grilled Fennel*

Dessert Fruit and Nut Bar*

Wednesday

Breakfast Steamed kale with garlic and lemon, topped with 3 eggs cooked in canola or flaxseed oil

Sliced strawberries

Hot tea

Lunch Gazpacho*

Spinach salad with grilled chicken, tomato, and cucumber

Glass of fresh-brewed iced tea

Snack Banana with trail mix of almonds, dried cranberries, and pumpkin seeds

Dinner Grilled salmon filet rubbed with orange zest, smoked paprika, and olive oil (serve atop a bed of spinach with orange wedges and roasted red pepper)

Glass of red wine (suggestion: Pinot Noir)

Thursday

Breakfast   Grilled salmon with steamed broccoli and topped with a dollop of plain Greek yogurt mixed with Everyday Chimichurri

Glass of orange juice

Lunch   Chopped salad with tomatoes, cucumbers, scallions, shredded carrots, and toasted cashews, tossed with Everyday Chimichurri

Snack   Watermelon slices

Dinner   Tuna Burger* served open-faced atop a French baguette

Sautéed bok choy and shiitake mushrooms topped with sesame seeds

Dessert   Scoop of fruit sorbet topped with chopped dark chocolate

Friday

Breakfast   Tuna burger topped with a poached egg

Spinach salad with shredded carrots, cabbage, and leftover Tuna Burger

Cup of coffee

Lunch   Roasted Sweet Potato and Poblano Salad with Grilled Chicken*

Fresh-brewed iced green tea with lemon wedges

Snack   ½ avocado sprinkled with lemon juice, ground walnuts, and flaxseeds

Dinner   Sirloin with Tangy Red Cabbage and Beets*

Parsnip-Apple Mash*

Dessert   3 Medjool dates, pitted and stuffed with almonds or Homemade Nut Butter*

Saturday

Breakfast   Sautéed shrimp with spinach, mushrooms, and garlic

1 cup grapes

Hot tea

Lunch   Potato salad made with mashed avocado in place of
             mayonnaise and topped with a sliced, hardboiled egg
             Orange slices

Snack   Apple

Dinner   Pork Tenderloin with Fig Sauce and Cauliflower Puree*
             Steamed Brussels sprouts, sautéed with walnut oil and
             garlic, sprinkled with chopped walnuts
             Glass of red wine (suggestion: Zinfandel)

Dessert   5 dried apricots dipped in melted dark chocolate

Sunday

Breakfast Smoothie with berries, 1 banana, spinach, ice cubes, and
             a dash of cinnamon (enough for 2 servings; freeze half)

Lunch   Curry-rubbed chicken with Mediterranean salad of
             chopped tomato, cucumber, kalamata olives, capers,
             fresh parsley, and lemon juice

Snack   Celery, carrot, and cucumber sticks sprinkled with
             lemon juice and curry powder

Dinner   Grilled Shrimp Skewers with Bell Peppers and
             Pineapple,* brushed with Universal Marinade
             Steamed or grilled asparagus
             Baked potato drizzled with extra-virgin olive oil

Dessert   Frozen smoothie (other half from breakfast)

Monday

Breakfast 3-egg omelet (discard 1 yolk) with asparagus, scal-
             lions, and Everyday Chimichurri
             Leftover potato, cubed and sautéed with canola oil and
             onions
             Honeydew melon and pineapple
             Cup of coffee

Lunch   Mixed greens salad with turkey, radish, green peppers,
             celery, and sunflower seeds, drizzled with balsamic
             vinegar and extra-virgin olive oil

Snack   Inner romaine lettuce leaves dipped in a mixture of
             mashed avocado, Everyday Chimichurri, and chopped
             tomato

Dinner   Ropa Vieja* Double the recipe to make enough for
             tomorrow's lunch, too.
             Mashed sweet potatoes with orange juice
             Glass of red wine (suggestion: Shiraz)

Dessert   Half grapefruit, drizzled with honey

Tuesday

Breakfast Portobello Egg Stack*
             Fruit salad
             Hot tea

Lunch   Ropa Vieja* served in collard greens or romaine leaves
             with fresh salsa and jalapeños
             Apple

Snack   Smoothie of your choice

Dinner   Honey Dijon halibut (Brush halibut fillets with a mix-
             ture of Dijon, honey, and cayenne pepper; sauté over
             medium-high heat until flaky, 6 to 8 minutes.)
             Sautéed zucchini and summer squash tossed with
             Everyday Chimichurri
             Glass of white wine (suggestion: Chardonnay or
             Sauvignon Blanc)

Dessert   1 ounce dark chocolate

Wednesday

Breakfast Salmon-egg salad with 1 cup flaked salmon (cold), 1
             diced, hard-boiled egg, chopped scallions, minced dill
             pickle, and extra-virgin olive oil over spinach leaves

Lunch   Pork tenderloin with Everyday Chimichurri over
             shaved fennel bulb**, carrot and onion salad tossed
             with Universal Marinade

Snack	Steamed green beans sprinkled with sesame seeds
Dinner	Rainbow Salad with Moroccan Spiced Chicken*
Dessert	Peach and/or pear

**Trim the stalks and cut off the very bottom of the bulb; then cut it in half lengthwise. Shave it on a mandolin or very thinly by hand.

Thursday

Breakfast	Pork tenderloin over sautéed baby bok choy ½ roasted sweet potato Sliced pineapple Cup of coffee
Lunch	2 hardboiled eggs topped with Everyday Chimichurri 1 orange
Snack	Ants on a Log (fill celery sticks with almond butter and top with raisins)
Dinner	Five-Spice Seared Scallops (dust with five-spice powder and sear 1½ to 2 minutes per side in canola oil over medium-high heat) Sautéed asparagus, red pepper, and garlic, tossed with curry paste, scallions, and a dash of soy sauce. Top with pumpkin seeds.
Dessert	Dried cherries and dark chocolate

Friday

Breakfast	Blueberries and strawberries "cereal" topped with Almond Milk* and chopped almonds
Lunch	Turkey tenderloin with raspberry salsa (chopped red onion, cucumber, jalapeño, and lime juice stirred with smashed raspberries) Bed of baby spinach leaves
Snack	Steamed brussels sprouts, sautéed in canola oil with garlic

Dinner	Mahi-mahi broiled with Everyday Chimichurri until flaky Steamed zucchini "pasta"** with garlic and tomatoes Mixed greens salad
Dessert	Cinnamon-baked apples with nuts (Halve and core the apple, sprinkle it with cinnamon, and place the halves in a glass dish with ½ inch of orange juice; bake covered for 20 to 30 minutes or until tender. Top with chopped nuts.)

**Slice off both ends and halve lengthwise, using a mandolin or slice carefully with a sharp knife into 1/8-inch slices to resemble pasta. Steam and toss with garlic and chopped tomatoes. Make enough for tomorrow's breakfast.

Saturday

Breakfast	Zucchini pasta with 2 poached eggs and chopped walnuts 2 plums Hot tea
Lunch	Ground veal or lamb sautéed with onions, garlic, and your favorite spices, served in collard green or Swiss chard leaves (save half for tomorrow) Sliced strawberries with fresh mint
Snack	Banana and raisins
Dinner	Baked tilapia with Universal Marinade and Everyday Chimichurri tartar sauce made with canola oil mayo Sautéed leeks** and green beans in canola oil with garlic Glass of white wine (suggestion: Dry Riesling or Pinot Grigio)
Dessert	Grilled pineapple with a small scoop of frozen vanilla yogurt sprinkled with chopped crystallized ginger (Grill the pineapple over medium heat until the grill marks show and the pineapple is warm, about 5 minutes total.)

**Trim the green tops and roots from the leeks. Cut them in half lengthwise and run them under cold water while fanning out the layers to rinse. Cut the leeks crosswise into moon-shaped ½-inch pieces, and sauté as if they were onion slices.

Sunday

Breakfast	Ground meat (from yesterday's lunch) mixed in with scrambled eggs and topped with Everyday Chimichurri Fresh berries Coffee with 1 teaspoon cocoa powder stirred in
Lunch	Cabbage, Cucumber, and Dill Salad*
Snack	Halved cherry tomatoes tossed with olive oil, balsamic vinegar, and basil
Dinner	Grilled chicken kabobs with mushrooms, onions, and cherry tomatoes, brushed with Everyday Chimichurri after grilling Mixed greens Glass of red wine
Dessert	Frozen banana with chocolate (Peel a banana, dip in melted dark chocolate, sprinkle with chopped nuts, and place on waxed paper; freeze until firm.)

Vitamin D Cure Recipes

Vitamin D Cure Everyday Chimichurri (EC)

Makes ½ cup.

½ cup loosely packed fresh parsley

½ cup loosely packed fresh basil leaves

3 tablespoons loosely packed herb of your choice: thyme, rosemary, dill, cilantro

1 tablespoon minced garlic

2 tablespoons water

1 tablespoon fresh lemon juice

¼ teaspoon fresh ground black pepper

2 tablespoons extra-virgin olive oil or canola oil

Combine all of the ingredients except the oil in a food processor and process until everything is finely minced.

While the machine is running, pour in the oil until it is well blended.

Vitamin D Cure Champagne Vinaigrette

Makes 1½ cups.

½ cup Champagne vinegar

1 tablespoon country-style Dijon mustard

2 cloves garlic, minced

1 teaspoon honey

1 cup extra-virgin olive oil or canola oil

Combine all of the ingredients in a jar with a tight-fitting lid; shake them to combine.

Vitamin D Cure Avocado Scramble Wrap

Makes 1 serving.

3 omega eggs

Small amount canola oil

½ avocado, diced

1 medium tomato, diced

Juice of ½ lemon

Steamed whole leafy greens (kale, mustard, Swiss chard, you name it!)

Sprouts (alfalfa, broccoli, or onion)

In a small pan, scramble 3 eggs in a small amount of canola oil.

Remove the pan from the heat. Gently stir in the avocado, tomato, and lemon juice.

Spoon the eggs into a whole leaf of the leafy green you prefer and top with sprouts.

Vitamin D Cure Homemade Nut Butter

Makes about 1 cup.

8 ounces dry-roasted nuts (almonds, pecans, walnuts, pistachios, etc.)
1 tablespoon canola or flaxseed oil (if needed)
1 tablespoon ground flaxseeds

In a food processor, grind the nuts until a paste forms. (Be patient. It takes a few minutes for the nuts to release the oils and turn into a paste form. With dry nuts such as almonds, you may need to add a small amount of oil.)

Once the butter is smooth, add the ground flaxseeds and pulse until they're incorporated.

Vitamin D Cure Balsamic Marinated Skirt Steak with Grilled Fennel

Makes 4 servings.

1 pound skirt steak, trimmed of fat
½ cup balsamic vinegar
¼ cup plus 2 tablespoons Everyday Chimichurri
2 fennel bulbs, stalks and bottom of bulb removed
Olive oil
Freshly ground pepper
Juice of ½ lemon

Combine the skirt steak with the balsamic vinegar and ¼ cup of Chimichurri. Let it sit for at least 30 minutes or overnight.

Cut the fennel bulbs in half lengthwise and then into 4 to 6 more wedges, trying to keep all of the layers intact at the bottom, so that they are as manageable as possible on the grill.

Brush the wedges with olive oil and season with freshly ground pepper.

Preheat the grill to medium-high heat.

Remove the steak from the marinade, let the excess drip off, and lightly pat the steak dry. Place it on the grill, turning it once, until it reaches the desired doneness (for a ½-inch thick steak, about 6 to 8 minutes total for medium-rare). Remove it from the grill and make a tent of aluminum foil over the top while the fennel grills.

Add the fennel wedges to the grill. Grill them for about 10 minutes, turning them once with tongs, until they have grill marks and are tender. Combine the lemon juice and remaining 2 table-spoons of Chimichurri and drizzle this over the grilled fennel.

Serve the fennel wedges with the steak.

Vitamin D Cure Fruit and Nut Bars

Makes 12 bars.

¼ cup orange, apple, or cranberry juice

5 dates, halved and pitted

1 cup whole almonds

¾ cup dried fruit (mix and match anything you have on hand: raisins, cherries, prunes, apricots, and so on)

¼ cup pumpkin seeds or walnuts

¼ cup sunflower seeds

Preheat the oven to 300 degrees Fahrenheit. Line a baking sheet with parchment paper.

Pour the juice over the dates and let them soak for at least 5 minutes, mashing them slightly with a fork.

In a food processor, add the almonds and dried fruit. Pulse a few times to coarsely chop the mixture. Next, add the soaked dates and continue pulsing until the mixture starts to stick together.

Add the last 2 ingredients and pulse a few more times just to incor-porate.

Using your wet hands, scoop the mixture onto a clean work surface and flatten the mixture into a square sheet, about ½-inch thick (don't worry too much about how they look because they will taste just the same). Cut the sheet into 12 bars.

Arrange the bars on the lined baking sheet and bake for 10 minutes. Flip and continue baking another 8 to 10 minutes or until the nuts start to toast and dry out. Remove the bars from oven and let them cool.

Store the bars in an airtight container.

Vitamin D Cure Gazpacho with Avocado

(In just 10 minutes!)

Makes 4 servings.

½ cucumber, diced (reserve ¼ cup for garnish)
½ bell pepper, diced
3 medium tomatoes (about 2½ cups chopped)
¼ cup chopped red onion
1 cup tomato juice, cold
1 tablespoon red wine vinegar
2 teaspoons extra-virgin olive oil
¼ teaspoon freshly ground pepper
1 avocado, cubed

In a food processor, combine the cucumber, pepper, tomatoes, and red onion; pulse until they're pureed.

Add the next 4 ingredients (through the ground pepper) and pulse a few more times to combine everything.

Remove the mixture from the food processor and stir in the cubed avocado.

Ladle the Gazpacho into bowls and top it with a cucumber garnish.

Vitamin D Cure Fresh Tuna Burgers

Makes 4 burgers.

For the sauce:
1 tablespoon fresh grated ginger
1 carrot, peeled and roughly chopped
2 tablespoons rice vinegar
1 tablespoon low-sodium soy sauce

1 tablespoon sesame oil

2 tablespoons water

For the burgers:

1 pound fresh tuna, cut into chunks

2 tablespoons extra-virgin olive oil

2 tablespoons low-sodium soy sauce

Juice of ½ lime

¼ cup fresh chopped cilantro

1 tablespoon fresh grated ginger

1 teaspoon sesame oil

Spicy sprouts, for garnish

In a food processor, pulse the ginger and carrot until they're minced. Next, add the remaining sauce ingredients except the water, and continue processing until the mixture is smooth.

Drizzle in 2 tablespoons of water to achieve a saucelike consistency; transfer this to a bowl and set it aside.

For the burgers, in the same food processor bowl add the tuna chunks. Pulse a few times to roughly chop the tuna.

In a separate bowl, combine the remaining burger ingredients (through the ginger) and then pour them over the tuna. Continue to process until everything is well blended.

Form the mixture into 4 burgers and brush them with 1 teaspoon of sesame oil.

Grill the burgers over medium-high heat until they reach the desired doneness (about 2 minutes on each side for rare).

Toss the sprouts in the sauce and top each burger with the mixture.

Vitamin D Cure Roasted Sweet Potato and Poblano Salad with Grilled Chicken

Makes 4 servings.

2 tablespoons honey

1½ tablespoons red wine vinegar

1 tablespoon fresh chopped rosemary

1 small shallot, minced

2 teaspoons Dijon mustard

¼ cup extra-virgin olive oil

For the salad:

2½ pounds red-skinned sweet potatoes, peeled and cut into 1-inch pieces

2 fresh poblano chiles, seeded and diced

A little more extra-virgin olive oil

2 chicken breasts, grilled and cut into 1-inch cubes

¼ cup thinly sliced scallions

¼ cup fresh chopped parsley

Preheat the oven to 425 degrees Fahrenheit.

Combine the first 5 dressing ingredients in a small bowl and whisk to combine them. Gradually whisk in the oil until it's combined.

Toss the cubed sweet potato and poblano chiles with a little olive oil, and spread the cubes in a single layer on a baking sheet. Roast them in a preheated oven 15 to 20 minutes or until tender. Remove them from the oven and let them cool to room temperature.

In a large bowl, combine the dressing, roasted potatoes, poblanos, grilled chicken, scallions, and fresh parsley. Gently toss to coat everything evenly with dressing, and serve the salad at room temperature.

Vitamin D Cure Beef with Tangy Red Cabbage and Beets

Make 4 servings.

3 tablespoons olive oil

¾ pound sirloin steak

1 teaspoon crushed caraway seeds

½ teaspoon black pepper

1 large onion, sliced

6 cups shredded red cabbage (about 1 medium head)

1 large beet, trimmed, peeled, and grated
¼ cup cider vinegar
1 tablespoon honey
¾ cup water
2 tablespoons fresh chopped dill

Heat the olive oil in a large skillet over high heat, and season the steak with caraway seeds and black pepper. Add the steak to the skillet and cook, turning it once, for 8 minutes for medium-rare. Transfer it to a cutting board and tent it with foil to keep it warm.

To the same skillet, add the sliced onion, and sauté for about 5 minutes. Add the cabbage and beet and cook another 5 minutes or until the cabbage is wilted. Add the vinegar, honey, and ¾ cup of water. Lower the heat to medium-low and cook, stirring often, until the cabbage is tender, about 10 minutes. Stir in the fresh dill.

Slice the steak against the grain, and add the accumulated juices to the cabbage. Serve the sliced steak atop the cabbage mixture.

Vitamin D Cure Parsnip-Apple Mash

Makes 4 servings.

1 pound parsnips, peeled and cut into same-size chunks
1 pound Fuji or Pink Lady apples, peeled, cored, and cut into chunks
1 cup vegetable broth
1 tablespoon olive oil or canola oil
Freshly ground black pepper

Combine the first 3 ingredients in a medium-size saucepan and bring everything to a boil. Reduce the heat, cover, and cook until the parsnips and apples are tender (about 25 minutes).

Transfer them to a food processor and blend until smooth, drizzling in olive oil while the motor is running.

Season the mash with black pepper and serve.

Vitamin D Cure Pork Tenderloin with Fig Sauce and Cauliflower Puree

Makes 4 servings.

2½ cups chicken or vegetable broth/stock

½ head cauliflower, cut into small florets

1 teaspoon paprika

¹/ teaspoon ground cinnamon

½ teaspoon dried thyme

¼ teaspoon ground black pepper

1 pork tenderloin, trimmed of fat

2 tablespoons olive oil

¼ cup balsamic vinegar

8 dried figs, stems removed and sliced

1 tablespoon fresh chopped thyme leaves

Preheat the oven to 400 degrees Fahrenheit. In a saucepan, bring 1½ cups of the broth or stock to a boil. Add the cauliflower and simmer until tender. With an immersion or standing mixer, puree the cauliflower until it's smooth.

In a small bowl, combine the rub ingredients (the paprika through the black pepper.) Coat the pork tenderloin evenly with the rub.

Heat the oil in a large sauté pan. Once the oil is hot, add the pork tenderloin; brown it on all sides. When it's evenly browned, transfer it to a baking sheet and finish it in the oven until the internal temperature reads 145 degrees. Let it rest 5 to 10 minutes and keep it warm.

Meanwhile, in the sauté pan, pour out the excess fat, and add the balsamic vinegar to deglaze by scraping the sides to get all of the browned bits from the pan. Cook this for 30 seconds, and add the remaining cup of broth or stock. Continue cooking it for 5 minutes or until it's reduced by half.

Stir in the figs and fresh thyme.

Slice the pork into 4 equal portions. Divide the cauliflower puree among four plates. Top it with the pork, and finish it with the fig sauce.

Vitamin D Cure Ropa Vieja

This traditional Cuban stew gets its name from the shredded meat that translates to "old clothes." It's delicious right out of the bowl and also perfect for tacos and burritos.

Makes 6–8 servings.

Small amount of olive oil
2 (1-pound) flank steaks, trimmed of excess fat
2 red onions, thinly sliced
2 each green and red peppers, sliced into strips
4 cloves garlic, minced
1 teaspoon dried oregano
1 teaspoon ground cumin
½ teaspoon dried crushed rosemary
½ teaspoon freshly ground black pepper
⅓ cup sherry vinegar
3 cups low-sodium beef broth or stock
1 tablespoon tomato paste (no-salt-added variety)
2 bay leaves
½ cup chopped fresh cilantro
Hot sauce

Heat a large Dutch oven over medium-high heat, and coat the bottom with olive oil. Add 1 steak to the pan and brown each side. Remove it and repeat with the other steak.

Reduce the heat slightly, and add the onions, peppers, and garlic; stirring regularly, sauté 6 to 8 minutes or until the vegetables are tender.

Stir in the next 4 ingredients, and cook for another 30 seconds or until the herbs and spices become fragrant. Stir in the vinegar, while scraping the pan to loosen the browned steak pieces; cook 1 to 2 minutes or until most of the liquid has evaporated.

Next, add the broth or stock, tomato paste, and bay leaves, and return the steaks to the pan (with the accumulated juices). Bring them to a simmer; cover, reduce the heat, and cook them

90 minutes or until the steaks are very tender and can be shredded apart with a fork.

Discard the bay leaves, and remove the steaks from the pan. Shred them with two forks, and return them to the pan. Add the cilantro, and ladle everything into bowls. Pass the hot sauce for a traditional fiery touch.

Vitamin D Cure Portobello Egg Stack

Makes 2.

2 Portobello mushroom caps, cleaned, with inner membrane scooped out

2 tablespoons extra-virgin olive oil

2 eggs

Universal Marinade

4 ounces spinach

2 large slices tomato

Preheat the grill or grill pan to medium-high heat. Brush the mushroom caps with oil and grill them for 6 to 8 minutes, turning once, until they're tender and grill-marked.

Meanwhile, prepare the eggs (poached, fried, or scrambled).

In a small sauté pan, add a small amount of Universal Marinade and wilt the spinach.

To assemble, place each mushroom cap with the underside facing up; fill it with the sautéed spinach. Next, layer the tomato slice, and top the stack with an egg. Drizzle the stacks with Universal Marinade.

Vitamin D Cure Rainbow Salad with Moroccan Spiced Chicken

Makes 2 large salads.

1 teaspoon ground cumin

1 teaspoon ground ginger

¼ teaspoon turmeric

¾ teaspoon black pepper

½ teaspoon ground cinnamon

½ teaspoon ground coriander

½ teaspoon cayenne

½ teaspoon ground allspice

¼ teaspoon ground cloves

2 chicken breasts, skinless and boneless

1 beet, peeled and diced

1 large carrot, shredded

1 avocado, diced

2 eggs, hardboiled, chopped or sliced

¼ cup dried cranberries

4 dates, pitted and chopped

¼ cup chopped almonds

1 sweet potato, cooked and diced

1 roasted red pepper, chopped

Champagne Vinaigrette (recipe on page 83)

Mixed greens

Preheat the grill to medium-high heat.

Combine the cumin through the cloves and whisk. Pat the chicken dry, and rub it evenly with the spice mixture. Grill the chicken for about 12 minutes, turning it once, or until it's no longer pink. Let it rest for 5 minutes.

In a large bowl, combine the remaining ingredients (except the mixed greens), and toss to combine.

Place the mixed greens on a plate and top with the salad mixture. Finish with the sliced chicken.

Vitamin D Cure Almond Milk

Makes 1 quart.

1 cup raw almonds

3 cups water

3 dates, pitted

1 teaspoon cinnamon (optional)

Combine the water and almonds; soak overnight.

In a blender, combine the almonds, water, and pitted dates (and cinnamon, if you like), and mix everything on high for 2 minutes.

Strain the mixture through a cheesecloth-lined strainer into a large bowl. Once all of it has strained through, discard the cheesecloth. Store the milk in a glass container in the refrigerator.

Serve it over berries or blend it into smoothies.

Vitamin D Cure Cabbage, Cucumber, and Dill Salad

Makes 4 servings.

$\frac{1}{4}$ cup lemon juice or white balsamic vinegar

2 tablespoons extra-virgin olive oil

1 teaspoon Dijon mustard

1 clove garlic, minced

$\frac{1}{2}$ head Napa or Savoy cabbage, shredded

4 scallions, thinly sliced

1 English cucumber, halved lengthwise and sliced

$\frac{1}{2}$ cup slivered almonds, toasted

2 tablespoons fresh chopped dill

In a large bowl, whisk the lemon juice or vinegar with the oil, Dijon, and garlic until everything is combined.

Add the remaining ingredients, and toss to coat the vegetables evenly.

Chill the salad for at least 2 hours to let the flavors meld.

Vitamin D Cure 2+2 Smoothies

Serves 1.

Smoothies are a great way to get water, fruit, and vegetables all in one glass. The smoothie I mix up tastes great, and I can make it in minutes. This is the perfect power refreshment for kids—or for anyone playing sports or exercising.

Smoothies also can make great salad dressings or dressings for meats.

2 fruits

2 vegetables

½ cup water or 100 percent fruit juice (orange, cranberry, apple, grapefruit—you choose)

½ cup sliced avocado (optional)

1. Select 2 fruits from the first column and 2 vegetables from the second column of the accompanying table.

2. Put 2 fruits and 2 vegetables in a food processor or a blender and blend.

3. Add ½ cup water or fruit juice (orange juice, cranberry juice, or another juice) to thin as needed, or use low-fat, unsweetened plain yogurt.

4. Don't add sugar; the fruit has sugar to sweeten the smoothie.

5. Add slices of avocado to the blender mixture for the creamiest smoothie ever.

Quick tip: Buy fresh baby spinach leaves, wash them, and freeze them in a large, sealed plastic bag. Once these are frozen, crush the leaves in the bag, and put them back in the freezer so you have handy frozen spinach flakes that you can add to smoothies or other dishes.

SOME 2+2 SMOOTHIE CHOICES	
Fruits	**Vegetables**
Apple slices	Baby carrots
Bananas	Broccoli florets
Blueberries	Cabbage, chopped
Kiwi slices	Celery, chopped
Orange wedges	Kale, chopped
Pear slices	Peppers, chopped
Plum slices	Spinach flakes
Strawberries	Zucchini slices

7

Step Four: Cover Your Bases with Other Supplements

Step Four maps out your complete supplementation plan. Setting this up is a giant step toward greater health, but it doesn't have to be complicated.

Here's a typical supplementation plan:

- Multivitamin and mineral supplement (as needed based on diet)
- Vitamin D supplement (see recommendations in chapter 5)
- Magnesium supplement
- Concentrated omega-3 fatty acid supplement

Don't forget that while you're popping these pills, you also need to eat good food or the picture will be incomplete.

Dietary changes can be tough to handle, but supplements are inexpensive insurance policies. They buy you some wiggle room with your diet as you tackle dietary challenges. Most of us fail to get enough of many important nutrients, and as you transition to a healthier eating plan, it makes good sense to supplement deficiencies until your diet provides what you need. Supplement the essential nutrients you're lacking. You can do this adequately and inexpensively while you're also upgrading your diet.

An inexpensive multivitamin and mineral supplement supplies many nutrients. Some nutrients, though, are too bulky to fit into a single pill, so you may need to take additional tablets or capsules to get those. I found that as my diet improved I did not need to take the multivitamin/mineral supplement every day. Currently I take it about once a week. Remember that these are supplements, not replacements for real food, sunlight, and exercise.

Nutrients You Need

Nutrients we lack reflect urban lifestyles. Typically, North Americans don't eat enough produce and fish; plus, we don't exercise outdoors as much as we should. So we are missing nutrients found in seafood, vegetables, and sunshine. Seafood is rich in B vitamins and omega-3 fatty acids. Colored veggies are loaded with potassium, magnesium, calcium, vitamin K, vitamin A, folic acid, and a number of other trace elements. Let's look at some of these key nutrients.

B_3 (Niacin), B_6 (Pyridoxine), B_9 (Folic Acid), B_{12} (Cyanocobalamin)

Lean meats, vegetables, and fruits have B vitamins. Fresh fish and other seafood have high concentrations of niacin and pyridoxine. Green leafy vegetables such as spinach and collards are good sources of folic acid. Clams, mussels, fish, grazing animals, and eggs have vitamin B_{12}.

Niacin is important in your diet because it facilitates DNA repair and may help reduce your risk of cancer. Niacin in high doses can lower total cholesterol and bad cholesterol (LDL) and raise good cholesterol (HDL), potentially reducing your risk of heart attack and stroke. Niacin also has potent anti-inflammatory actions that independently account for some of its prevention of cardiovascular disease.

Pyridoxine, folic acid, and vitamin B_{12} are extremely important in the new science of epigenetics. These B vitamins modify DNA (methylation), altering the expression of genes. These modifications of DNA caused by more or less methylation can be passed on for several generations. This may determine your risk for obesity and diabetes—and the risk of future generations (see chapter 9). As bizarre as it seems, what you ate as a child might actually affect the health of your great-grandchildren.

Folic acid is vital to fetal development and nervous system function, which makes it essential for the good health of pregnant women and young children. And, vitamin D appears to increase folic acid uptake into cells. Furthermore, depression and dementia in older adults have been linked to deficiencies of folic acid, vitamin B_6 and vitamin B_{12}.

Contrary to popular belief, refined grains don't contain many of these important nutrients. To make flour-based products seem more nutritious, many manufacturers add B vitamins to the mix when processing grains. What's better for your health, though, is bypassing cereals in favor of fresh seafood, lean meats, and vegetables.

As you can see, B vitamins influence many of the same biological systems as vitamin D, which shows the interconnected nature of nutrients. Take a multivitamin that contains 50 to 100 percent of your DRI for vitamins $B_{3, 6, 9,}$ and $_{12,}$ but avoid daily vitamins that provide 200 percent or more of these nutrients unless you're targeting a disease or a deficiency.

Vitamin D

You know that you can't get enough vitamin D from your diet, which means you need sun and supplements. Because foods such as dark-meat fish and organ meat provide only a minuscule amount of vitamin D, it's a good idea to follow the recommendations in chapters 4 and 5 to meet your vitamin D needs.

Vitamin K

Fat-soluble vitamin K is important for bones and blood vessels. High intakes of K reduce the risk of osteoporotic fracture and regulate bone mineralization.

If you're on blood thinners, you probably already know that vitamin K interferes with the action of blood thinners, but that doesn't mean that K causes blood to clot. On the contrary, you need adequate vitamin K to prevent blood clots. The factors in your blood that are most sensitive to vitamin K are your natural blood thinners that prevent blood from clotting.

You can get plenty of K from green, leafy vegetables such as spinach, kale, Swiss chard, and bok choy. Tea, especially green tea, is rich in vitamin K. Make sure to take a daily multivitamin that contains 75 to 100 percent (80 to 120 micrograms) of your DRI for vitamin K.

Potassium

Your body needs potassium to maintain acid-base balance, strengthen bones, and lower blood pressure, and the best source of potassium is food. Vegetables, fruits, and fresh seafood contain potassium, but grain-based foods have very little. Because it's impractical to try to supplement your way to enough potassium, eating plenty of vegetables and fruits is a far better plan.

Magnesium

Magnesium plays a key role in neutralizing acid from protein metabolism, and you need magnesium for more than three hundred enzymatic reactions. Just as important is that you need magnesium for proper functioning of vitamin D, PTH (parathyroid hormone), and calcitonin—three hormones that regulate bone metabolism and your mineral stores.

You absorb 30 to 50 percent of the magnesium that's in nuts, dried fruit, and green, leafy vegetables. Supplements, in contrast, allow you to absorb only about 5 to 15 percent of magnesium, and that's a two- to fourfold difference. A daily multiple vitamin can't contain adequate magnesium because it would be too large to swallow. Even multiple vitamin packets don't contain enough magnesium.

Other drawbacks are that magnesium supplements are poorly absorbed, and that unabsorbed magnesium draws water into your intestines and causes diarrhea. This makes it nearly impossible to develop magnesium toxicity unless you have kidney failure. You would have to consume about three times the amount of magnesium that causes diarrhea for it to become toxic. It's clear that you need to eat your way to sufficient magnesium stores for your body; the problem is that the food approach won't work if you follow a typical North American diet.

If you want to supplement, you can take two magnesium tablets a day (roughly 500 milligrams of any preparation), and increase the dose of magnesium by one tablet a day each week until you develop loose stools. When you get cramping or diarrhea, reduce your tablet intake by one tablet per day and stick with that level of supplementation. If six tablets a day give you loose bowels, cut back to five or fewer and stay there. This method effectively maximizes the amount of magnesium you can tolerate. As your stores replenish and your diet changes, you may absorb less, leading to loose stools again. If so, just cut the dose back again.

This method also reduces the confusion associated with choosing a magnesium preparation and figuring out how much elemental magnesium there is in different preparations. Typically, the best-absorbed alkaline forms are chelated magnesium such as magnesium citrate. With one of these, you probably can take more magnesium before you experience loose bowels.

A simpler way to supplement magnesium is to calculate your daily need based on Institute of Medicine (IOM) requirements and take that full amount as a supplement. This will ensure that you meet at least 15 percent of your magnesium requirement. The IOM estimates that a child needs magnesium of about 5 milligrams per kilogram of lean body mass per day. This translates to 2.3 milligrams per pound of lean body mass per day. For adults, the amount is 6 milligrams per kilogram of lean body mass, or 2.7 milligrams per pound of lean body mass. So, a 155-pound person needs about 420 milligrams of magnesium each day.

Omega-3 Fatty Acids

Omega-3 fatty acids are polyunsaturated fatty acids (PUFAs). They include linolenic acid (LNA), found in high concentrations in purslane, a green, leafy vegetable, and flaxseed. Eicosapentanoic acid (EPA) and docosahexanoic acid (DHA) are the animal omega-3 fats in fish and fish oils and organ meat.

DHA is your brain's dominant fatty acid; it makes up about 40 percent of the fat in your brain. In research studies, higher levels of DHA and EPA have been associated with a lower incidence of high blood pressure, heart disease, diabetes, depression, attention deficit disorder, and dementia. Omega-3 fats also improve insulin sensitivity.

More important, polyunsaturated fats bind to a variety of nuclear receptors and behave like hormones (cortisol, estrogen, vitamin D). In other words, both omega-6 and omega-3 fats influence what your genes do, right along with vitamin D and other steroid hormones. This is why diet has such a tremendous impact on your health.

Unfortunately, the typical North American diet has one of the lowest intakes of omega-3 fatty acids in the industrialized world—fewer than 200 milligrams a day. You get DHA when you eat dark-meat fish such as salmon, tuna, mackerel, and sardines (the very same kinds of fish that are high in vitamin D). Raw fish, such as sushi, is an even better source than cooked fish.

When primitive man consumed brain tissue from wild animals, he got generous amounts of DHA. Of course, the contamination of today's domesticated animal stocks with mad cow disease and other maladies has eliminated the option of eating animal brain and nervous tissue as sources of DHA. But wild game, organic beef, and grass- and pasture-fed animals have meats with more omega-3 fat than other meats available today. Many vegetarians supplement with DHA produced from microalgae.

Studies that show the benefits of omega-3 fatty acid supplementation typically start with about 2,000 to 3,000 milligrams of combined DHA and EPA per day. The FDA approved a commercially available omega-3 fatty acid supplement (Lovaza, Reliant Pharmaceuticals, Inc.)

at doses of 2,000 to 4,000 milligrams per day for treatment of high blood triglyceride levels.

You can supplement omega-3 fats with fish oils, but fish liver oils also contain significant amounts of vitamin A. Although vitamin A is important, in industrialized societies where people typically have access to good foods, vitamin A is not a limiting nutrient in diets. In addition, your daily multiple vitamin probably contains 100 percent of the DRI of vitamin A, so you want to avoid duplication and possible toxicity.

Fish oil supplements have only about 30 percent omega-3 by weight. This means that a 1,000-milligram gelcap of fish oil has only about 300 milligrams of omega-3 fat. In other words, to get 3,000 milligrams, you would have to take ten gelcaps a day. So look for concentrated omega-3 fatty acid supplements, usually labeled "Max EPA" or "Max DHA" or "Double or Triple Strength Fish Oil." These products are purified from fish oil using vacuum molecular distillation and have 50 to 80 percent omega-3 fat by weight. Concentrated forms have negligible amounts of vitamins A and D.

In studies of adults, researchers have seen no adverse effects with doses of up to 8,000 milligrams per day of combined EPA and DHA. A weight-based dose to achieve 2,000 milligrams a day in an average healthy adult would be about 15 milligrams per pound of body weight per day of combined EPA and DHA.

Calcium

Many vitamin D supplements contain calcium, and some also contain magnesium. Typically, such supplements don't have more than 200 IUs of vitamin D per tablet, which reduces their usefulness as a vitamin D supplement.

Most people are deficient in vitamin D, not in calcium. But remember that when your vitamin D level drops below 20 nanograms per milliliter, your need for dietary calcium doubles. To break even, you need to *absorb* about 300 milligrams of calcium, according to U.S. calculations on Americans.

The average American who is deficient in vitamin D and who has an acidic diet low in magnesium and potassium will need a daily supplement of 1,000 to 1,200 milligrams of calcium. You'll be able to absorb about 25 percent—300 milligrams, in other words—but you'll lose most of this calcium in urine and feces, so you break even.

According to studies by Dr. Robert Heaney of Creighton University, when your vitamin D level is 35 nanograms per milliliter or more, your efficiency of active calcium absorption hits its maximum at 30 to 40 percent. Below a vitamin D level of 20 nanograms per milliliter, this efficiency drops by 50 percent. But in studies of diverse populations, researchers find that average vitamin D levels lie between these two numbers. Raising your D levels may conservatively decrease your calcium needs by 25 to 50 percent, depending on how deficient you are.

Remember, too, that a diet with acid excess and lots of salt makes you lose calcium in your urine. This kind of loss can amount to 100 milligrams of calcium per day. If you absorb just 25 percent of dietary calcium when you're D deficient, you must take in 400 milligrams of calcium (four times as much as the loss) to balance this increased urinary loss.

Adjust your calcium needs based on normalizing your vitamin D levels and correcting your acid-base imbalance, and your calcium needs drop from 1,000 to 1,200 milligrams per day to 400 to 600. The typical American takes in about 600 to 900 milligrams of calcium, according to the 1999–2000 National Health and Nutrition Examination Survey (NHANES).

Magnesium supplementation and exercise further reduce calcium losses. In the end, you probably won't need calcium supplements at all if you normalize your vitamin D, balance the acid base in your diet, supplement magnesium, and regularly exercise.

In the meantime, until you know that you've gotten your D up to par, supplement your calcium at 500 to 600 milligrams per day. Once your vitamin D level is normal and your diet is on track, you can decrease your calcium supplementation further or eliminate it altogether.

If you eat six or more servings of produce a day, particularly green, leafy vegetables high in magnesium and calcium, supplementation isn't necessary. If you eat one or more servings of yogurt or skim milk a day and normalize your vitamin D, calcium supplementation isn't necessary. But if you have trouble sticking to the ratio of three times as much produce as protein, continue to take both magnesium and calcium supplements.

Don't take more than 600 milligrams of calcium per day if you're following the vitamin D supplementation guidelines in this book. Too much calcium supplementation can cause constipation and back pain, and recent studies show it may increase your risk of kidney stones, heart attacks, and strokes.

Knowing What to Take

You can refer to the following chart for supplement recommendations. The middle column lists current DRI recommendations. On the right are my recommendations, based on analysis and interpretation of today's best nutrition studies and my own hands-on experience with patients who improved their health via the Vitamin D Cure.

You can find a multivitamin that has the right amounts of many nutrients, but a daily vitamin won't have adequate amounts of vitamin D, magnesium, and omega-3 fatty acids. So to get appropriate amounts of these, you need to take additional supplements.

Use caution when taking supplements designed to target specific diseases or systems. These supplements can overlap with each other and your multivitamin/mineral, thus providing excessive and possibly unsafe amounts of specific nutrients. Minerals aren't easily eliminated and can accumulate in tissues, especially bone, producing toxicity. To avoid over-supplementation, create a chart that shows what each supplement contains and how much and how often you take it.

	THE VITAMIN D CURE DAILY RECOMMENDED INTAKES ALL SOURCES	
Nutrient	**2010 DRI/RDA**	**The Vitamin D Cure**
Vitamin A	3000 IU	2000 IU retinol or 7200 IU beta-carotene
Vitamin B$_3$	11–12 mg	20 mg
Vitamin B$_6$	1.3–1.4 mg	2.0 mg
Folate (B$_9$)	400 mcg	400 mcg
Vitamin B$_{12}$	2.4 mcg	3.0 mcg (age > 50, 10–30% malabsorb)
Vitamin C	75-90 mg	120 mg
Vitamin D	600 IU	20–25 IU/lb ABW (actual body weight)
Vitamin E	22 IU	40 IU (do not exceed 200 IU/d)
Vitamin K	120 mcg	120 mcg
Magnesium	320–420 mg	2.5 mg/lb IBW (ideal body weight)
Calcium	1000–1200 mg	0–600 mg
Omega 3	2 servings fish/wk	15–20 mg/lb IBW combined EPA + DHA

8

Step Five: Add a Little Exercise

Step Five—exercise—is an important part of the Vitamin D Cure. To work exercise into your lifestyle, try these things:

- Commit a thirty-minute block of time to daily exercise.
- Do daily stretches and strength exercises.
- Do cardio exercise thirty minutes three times a week.
- Meditate while you exercise.

Once you've corrected your vitamin D level and rebalanced your diet, you probably will have newfound energy that will come in handy when you add another key facet to your health upgrade: regular exercise.

The key is finding a protected time slot. Choose a thirty-minute block of time that is all yours. For many people, that's first thing in the morning or just before bedtime at night.

All you have to do is commit to protecting this time slot for exercise. Then you can also find other ways to fit exercise into your daily lifestyle:

walking in malls, strolling with a friend, taking your pets to the park. I do a thirty-minute block between six and six-thirty each morning. My commute is fifteen minutes, and I don't have to be at the office until seven forty-five, so this gives me ninety minutes to exercise, eat, and get ready for work.

You may wonder: why bother with exercise if you're doing all of the other important Vitamin D Cure steps? Here's why.

Vitamin D Boosts Your Exercise Benefits

Vitamin D helps you exercise better, longer, and more productively— you get better results, and your muscles work more efficiently, have more oomph, and are stronger.

There's a reciprocal relationship between D and exercise. Vitamin D improves exercise capacity for these reasons:

- Vitamin D preserves muscle mass.
- Vitamin D improves muscle performance.
- Exercise improves vitamin D production and supply.

We define exercise capacity in strength, coordination, and endurance. Strength is related to lean muscle mass—the more mass you have, the more strength you have. Coordination requires that small and large muscles fire rapidly and in controlled bursts to perform delicate or precise maneuvers. This control requires adequate numbers of nerves attached to your muscles, as well as well-tuned muscles that can contract and relax rapidly, with no muscle spasms or cramps.

Endurance requires optimal muscle metabolism, a healthy heart, and healthy lungs. Your muscle must be able to burn a variety of fuels efficiently, and the heart and lungs have to deliver enough oxygen to the muscle so it can burn that fuel.

Vitamin D Helps You Get the Job Done

Muscle mass is directly related to vitamin D, as well as to other variables, such as adequate protein. The severe vitamin D deficiency of osteomalacia and rickets results in muscle atrophy and weakness. These problems can be so severe that toddlers and adults lose their ability to walk; but replacing vitamin D restores their strength and coordination.

Stamina also is important in workouts. How long you can sustain repeated muscle contractions depends on the efficiency and supply of your fuel. Vitamin D improves insulin sensitivity, and this serves muscles well during exercise.

You need vitamin D to breathe well. Researchers measured how much air you can blow out in one second and the total amount of air you can blow out *period*, and they found that both were significantly higher in people with the highest vitamin D levels compared to those with the lowest levels. The differences were greatest in people sixty or older. The difference due to vitamin D was also greater than the difference due to smoking.

To get plenty of oxygen to your muscles during exercise, you need a strong heart and healthy blood vessels. Vitamin D lowers blood pressure and opens up your blood vessels, allowing more blood to flow.

Exercise Boosts Your Vitamin D

How does exercise enhance vitamin D? When you go outside to walk, bike, run, or row, you're exposed to sunlight, which facilitates vitamin D production. This increased production of D affects the production of collagen in skin, the growth of sweat glands, hair follicle life-cycles, and muscle and bone. The positive effects of sufficient vitamin D on hair follicles and sweat glands enhance your cooling efficiency during exercise.

The fuel burned during exercise varies with the type of exercise. During short, quick activities such as sprinting and power lifting, the body uses glucose. But during aerobic exercise or prolonged exertion, you primarily burn fat, and that's why aerobic exercise is so important for restoring and maintaining lean body mass. That's also the reason that aerobic exercise raises vitamin D levels. When you burn fat, you liberate vitamin D from that fat and garner it for use elsewhere. It's safe to attribute at least part of the health benefits of exercise to these higher vitamin D levels.

How much exercise does it take to burn fat? About 35 to 50 percent of your maximum oxygen-burning capacity (VO_2 max), which correlates with 50 to 65 percent of your maximum heart rate (MHR), is how hard you have to work to burn fat (see page 115). Much more or much less and your fat-burning drops off.

Furthermore, your efficiency at burning fat peaks at forty-five minutes, at about 60 percent MHR, and remains at that peak for another forty-five minutes before it begins to decline. The more often you exercise at 50 to 65 percent MHR for fifteen minutes or longer, the more efficient you become at burning fat, the more fat you burn, and the more vitamin D you liberate.

Exercise and diet also work together to direct nutrients where you need them. Working out pulls nutrients into your bones and muscles. The more muscle mass and bone mass you create, the more buffers (protein, potassium, magnesium, and calcium) you have for the following:

- balancing your acid-base
- running marathons
- surviving illnesses such as pneumonia or cancer

Exercise is like a shield that protects you from physical and biochemical stress. In addition, the more fat-free muscle you create with exercise, the higher your resting energy consumption. You burn more calories at rest when you have a greater amount of lean muscle.

On the flip side, inactivity leads to muscle atrophy and loss of muscle mass—or lower resting energy consumption. Inactivity wreaks all kinds of havoc by

- promoting the storage of energy as fat, which produces inflammatory substances;
- contributing to insulin resistance; and
- increasing physical stresses on your bones, joints, and cardiovascular system.

The Vitamin D Cure No-Sweat Workout

Here's an exercise routine that's simple, quick, and gets the job done without muss or fuss. Go to www.thevitamindcure.com to download the exercise video.

Stretches for Hip Extensors and Knee Flexors

You use these muscles every day for walking, rising from a sitting position, and climbing stairs. They are the strongest muscles in your body, and they get tighter as you age and become less active. They are the most common cause of pain in the buttocks and the pain called "sciatica." Stretching these muscles helps eliminate aches and pains.

Materials: Doorway or archway, floor

1. Lie on the floor with your hip bone next to the doorjamb or arch. Your body is positioned through the arch or doorway, legs perpendicular to the wall. Alternatively, lie with your legs parallel to the wall.

2. Lift your leg that's closer to the doorjamb and place the heel of your foot on the doorjamb.

3. Straighten your elevated knee and make sure your other leg is flat on the floor.

4. If you're not flexible enough to do this exercise, move your buttocks away from the doorjamb so that your butt aligns below your hip bone and toward the middle of your thigh. Repeat steps 2 and 3.

5. Remain in the stretched position 2 to 3 minutes.

6. Rotate your butt on the floor so that your opposite leg is now in position to stretch. Repeat steps 2 through 5.

Precautions: If you have a knee or hip replacement, review this stretch with your physical therapist or physician before trying it.

Push-Ups: Pain Relief for the Neck and Shoulder Area

Most people think of push-ups as a way to build pecs (chest muscles), and they will. But the hidden benefit is what push-ups can do for your neck and your back between your shoulder blades. As you do push-ups, you suspend your neck and thoracic spine. You may hear and feel cracks and pops while you're doing push-ups. But despite the sound effects, these exercises can reduce the pain in your neck and between your shoulder blades.

Material: Floor, carpeted

Option 1: Hands and Feet Planted

1. Roll onto your stomach with your legs straight out, hands closed in fists; plant your knuckles down into the carpet at chest level.
2. Turn your head to the right and hold that position.
3. Push up until your elbows are fully extended.
4. Let yourself down slowly until your chest muscles are stretched tight. Repeat this step for 1 minute.
5. Turn your head to the left and hold that position. Repeat steps 3 and 4.

Option 2: Hands and Knees Planted

1. Roll onto your hands and knees with your legs bent and your ankles crossed. Close your hands into fists and plant your knuckles fist down into the carpet at chest level.
2. Turn your head to the right and hold that position.
3. Push up until your elbows are fully extended. Then let yourself down slowly until your chest muscles are stretched tight. Repeat this step for 1 minute.
4. Turn your head to the left and hold that position. Repeat step 3.

Strengthening Hip Flexors: A Better Sit-Up for Back Pain

Low-back pain—so common that we all know someone who's troubled by it—is usually caused by one or more of these three things:

- Muscle problems (pulls, strains, etc.)
- Vitamin D deficiency
- Dietary imbalance

The most important muscles attached to your lower back are your hip flexors, which are responsible for the normal arch of your lower back. That's one reason why strengthening your hip flexors will do wonders for your lower-back pain.

The sit-up is for your back; abdominal muscles aren't going to make your back feel better. The key to doing sit-ups is to use your hip flexors more than your stomach muscles. As you pull yourself to a seated position, think about pulling your knees to your chest using your hip muscles. This is actually easier to do than using your stomach muscles. People who can't get up and down from the floor easily can strengthen their hip flexors while standing up.

Materials: Couch or table and ankle weights

Option 1: Lying Down

1. Lie down on the floor and hook your feet under the corner of a couch.
2. Position your buttocks so your knees are bent only about 20 degrees.
3. Put your hands at your ears or clasp them behind your neck.
4. Now pull yourself up to a seated position, using your hip flexors.
5. Slowly repeat this over and over for 5 minutes.
6. To kick it up a notch, pull one leg from under the couch, bend the leg with your foot on the floor, or cross it underneath the other knee. Now you're pulling with one set of hip flexors. Alternate sides halfway through.

Option 2: Standing Up

1. Stand beside a kitchen table or countertop. Balance by putting your hand that's nearer the surface atop the table or countertop.

2. Raise your right knee using your hip flexors above the level of your waist. Pause at the top.

3. Straighten your knee and lower your leg at the same time until your leg is back on the floor.

4. Repeat steps 2 and 3 with your left leg.

5. Continue to alternate legs for 5 minutes.

6. To kick it up a notch, strap on 5- to 10-pound ankle weights.

Dips for Shoulders and Arms to Ease Standing Up

One of the most common shoulder problems is arthritis in the joint where collarbone meets shoulder blade. As your rotator cuff weakens with age and lack of use over time, the ball joint tends to drift up into the shoulder. Combine this underuse and weakness with arthritis and you develop "impingement." But strengthening your rotator cuff can reduce the symptoms of impingement and may facilitate favorable remodeling of the joint when you normalize your vitamin D level and balance your diet.

Material: Sturdy coffee table or chair with arms

1. Sit on the edge of your coffee table. Place your hands at the edge.

2. Extend your feet in front of you, with your knees slightly bent.

3. Push up with your shoulders and arms until your elbows are fully extended, and slide your buttocks over the edge.

4. Relaxing your shoulders and bending at the elbow, let yourself down about 6 to 10 inches and then push back up until your elbows are extended.

5. Repeat step 4 for 1 minute without stopping.

6. To kick it up a notch, buy an exercise band and work the other elements of your rotator cuff.

The Final Stretches

The last stretch of the workout is intended for legs and shoulders—muscles that get tight when you sit for prolonged periods. Stretching your calves may help you reduce foot and heel pain when you're also improving your diet and vitamin D level. Stretching your thigh muscles helps to "unload" the knee for those of you who get pain behind the kneecap after a long period of sitting. The final stretch also just feels good.

Stretching Your Calves

1. Stand facing a wall, about 2 feet away from the wall.
2. Lean against the wall; move your right leg about 2 feet farther out from the wall.
3. Lean on the wall to apply pressure to your back leg, heel planted. You should feel a stretch in the right calf.
4. Hold the stretch for a count of 30.
5. Repeat this with your left leg.

Stretching Your Thigh Muscles

1. Standing next to the wall, place your right hand on the wall for balance.
2. Bend your right knee, moving your foot toward your buttocks.
3. Using your left hand, reach back and grab your right foot by the toes.
4. Standing up as straight as you can, pull on the right foot until you feel a stretch on the front of your thigh.
5. Hold the stretch for a count of 30.
6. Repeat for the left thigh.

Stretching Your Shoulders

1. Reach toward the ceiling with your right arm; hold this stretch for a count of 30.
2. Reach toward the ceiling with your left arm; hold this stretch for a count of 30.

Cardio Up for Better Health

When you hear people talk about getting in some cardio, they're referring to aerobic or cardiovascular exercise. Treadmill or elliptical machines may come to mind, and there's nothing wrong with either one, but you also can walk, bike, or swim. The point is, make sure you get aerobic three times a week, monitoring your heart rate or breathing to see that you're getting aerobic benefits.

It takes at least 12 minutes at an aerobic rate to reap the benefits of increased lean muscle mass and improved cardiovascular fitness. And if you want to lose weight and keep it off, you have to crank it up to at least 45 minutes of moderately intense aerobic exercise three or more times a week to build enough muscle mass to lower your set point.

The formula for calculating your training heart rate is as follows:

220 – age (years) = maximum heart rate (MHR)

15 to 20 minutes at (50 to 65 percent) MHR for maintenance fitness

45 minutes at (50 to 65 percent) MHR for weight loss

You can measure your own heart rate or use a heart rate monitor (about $40). A monitor stores the training heart rate you program in and beeps when you've reached your fitness zone and when you're above or below this zone. It also will track how much time you spend in the zone and beep at a preset duration of time in the zone. A heart rate monitor is a handy tool for monitoring your workouts.

If you can sing "Row, row, row your boat" and get all the way to "Merrily, merrily, merrily" before taking a breath, you're not exercising hard enough. If you can't get through "Row, row, row your boat" before taking a breath, your intensity is too high and you need to slow down. This is only an approximation, but you can use it to help keep you on track.

FIND YOUR FITNESS ZONE

Age	MHR	50% MHR	65% MHR
20	200	100	130
30	190	95	124
35	185	93	120
40	180	90	117
45	175	88	114
50	170	85	111
55	165	83	107
60	160	80	104
65	155	78	101
70	150	75	98
75	145	73	94
80	140	70	91
85	135	68	88
90	130	65	85

Mantra Your Way through Workouts

If you like multitasking, you can get double value from exercise time by adding in some meditation. Take this time as a perfect opportunity to relax and clear your mind of negative thoughts.

You can create your own mantra. Here's the one I say with each breath during my exercise routine:

I am not this body. (breath)

I am not this mind. (breath)

I am not my stuff. (breath)

I am infinite. (breath)

No expectations. (breath)

No judgments. (breath)

Only gratitude. (breath)

Enjoy!

PART THREE

The Vitamin D Cure for Total Health

Vitamin D deficiency causes disease. In part three, we spotlight:

- [ ] The metabolic syndrome—obesity, high blood pressure, diabetes, and heart disease
- [ ] The importance of vitamin D and diet for a healthy brain
- [ ] The influence of vitamin D and diet on your immune system function
- [ ] How vitamin D and diet fight cancer
- [ ] How vitamin D and diet regulate the health of your bones, joints, and teeth

Each of the next five chapters outlines the roles vitamin D deficiency and dietary imbalances play in causing disease. Examples and explanations of the latest science back up all contentions.

In chapter 9, you discover how vitamin D regulates your appetite and metabolism, lowering your risk of diabetes and heart disease. What you eat helps determine your metabolic set point. Chapter 10 explains how vitamin D deficiency can make you tired and can contribute to trouble with focus and memory. Chapters 11 and 12 shed light on the crucial roles vitamin D plays in allowing your immune system to recognize the difference between the bacteria in your nose and pneumonia—and how it identifies and fights cancer. Chapter 13 offers information on vitamin D's role in building bone and how a lack of vitamin D contributes to the development of arthritis.

Part three puts the Vitamin D Cure into perspective and helps motivate you to get started on your journey to better health.

9

The Vitamin D Cure for Obesity, High Blood Pressure, Diabetes, and Heart Disease

The metabolic syndrome is the constellation of obesity, high blood pressure, insulin resistance, and cardiovascular disease. Vitamin D deficiency is associated with important changes in metabolism that drive these diseases. Vitamin D deficiency

- increases the storage of energy as abdominal fat and decreases muscle mass;
- increases several stress hormones (renin and angiotensin), which raise blood pressure;
- decreases insulin release and insulin sensitivity in the muscle;
- facilitates inflammation that can damage blood vessels.

119

The balance of protein to produce in your diet, or your acid-base balance, can change many hormonal mechanisms. The chronic metabolic acid-base imbalance that comes from too much salt, cheese, and grain causes many of the same changes that acidosis from other diseases generates. They create a "stress response" that

- increases production and release of cortisol;
- reduces growth hormone production and function;
- decreases the efficient function of thyroid hormone;
- increases release of renin, angiotensin, aldosterone, and adrenaline;
- increases PTH release in response to low calcium; and
- increases the activation of vitamin D.

These hormonal changes

- accelerate bone turnover and mobilize protein and minerals from the musculoskeletal system;
- increase abdominal fat stores, further lowering vitamin D levels;
- raise blood pressure, bad cholesterol (LDL), and triglycerides;
- stimulate an inflammatory response; and
- produce insulin resistance.

Over time, all of these changes can increase your risk of heart attack, stroke, and diabetes.

The nutrients you eat regulate your metabolism and determine how well it works. A diet high in magnesium—an alkaline mineral—improves insulin sensitivity and glucose control. Saturated fats and simple carbohydrates, on the other hand, make you store energy as fat and reduce your insulin sensitivity. Omega-3 fatty acids stop fat production and improve insulin sensitivity. What you eat runs your metabolism.

The combination of obesity, high blood pressure, diabetes, and cardiovascular disease—commonly called "the metabolic syndrome"—is clearly a lifestyle disease, but many people wonder when environmental factors actually influence the development of disease. The answer is from the beginning of your life.

You Control Your Epigenome

You experience the most impact from vitamin D deficiency and lifestyle at conception and during fetal development, so a significant part of the risk for developing metabolic syndrome occurs in the uterus when the fetus is growing. Specifically, Dr. David Barker of Oregon Health and Science University has shown that nutritional stress at this early stage of development can permanently change our risk for these diseases. Animal studies confirm that inadequate fetal nutrition affects the development of the liver, pancreas, brain, kidneys, bones, and muscles.

When a developing fetus fails to get vital nutrients, development adapts to the scarcity, resulting in smaller kidneys and different profiles of liver enzymes. These adaptations predispose that baby to develop problems such as high blood pressure and diabetes or high cholesterol in adulthood.

The name for environmental influence on gene expression is epigenetics. This means that factors such as diet, emotions good and bad, stress, and exercise can all establish the pattern of your gene expression without changing the gene sequence. These lifestyle factors are as important as genes and in many cases more important than the genes themselves—and you control the influence.

The new patterns of gene expression can be passed on to your children and grandchildren. In fact, it may take several generations to wash out the effects of dietary stress and/or chemical exposure. Vitamin D has the ability to produce some of these epigenetic effects. For example, your mother's vitamin D level during pregnancy in part predicts the strength of your bones later in childhood and probably in late adulthood.

What this tells us is that we have both genetic-based risk and fetal-environmental-based risk—the old nature-versus-nurture issue. What we didn't know until recently is that the most important part of nurture begins at conception, not at birth.

You can't change history, so that just makes your current lifestyle even more pivotal. The truth is, if you have a high risk for disease and health problems, you need to be well disciplined about maintaining a healthy lifestyle—and you also may need medications to control those risk factors.

If you're obese, your body is sending your nutrients to fat storage, and that's the wrong place. The more fat you have stored, the more momentum you have for storage because your vitamin D levels are lower and your fat cells produce inflammatory substances that make you more resistant to insulin and leptin. Obesity makes you resistant to brain signals that would otherwise decrease your appetite by telling you "enough."

Vitamin D deficiency also depletes muscle, which reduces your fat-burning machinery and worsens insulin resistance. Acid excess in the diet promotes the hormonal changes that lead to obesity. But normalizing vitamin D and neutralizing diet acid can break this cycle.

Fighting the Metabolic Syndrome

If you have three or more of the following, you have metabolic syndrome.

- Big waist (waist size: more than 40 inches in men; more than 35 inches in women)
- Elevated blood triglycerides: 150 or more
- Low HDL (good cholesterol): men, lower than 40; women, lower than 50
- Elevated blood pressure, more than 130/85
- High blood glucose: fasting, 110 or more

For more statistics and information on the metabolic syndrome, see www.nlm.nih.gov/medlineplus/metabolicsyndromex.html.

The Truth about Being Fat

Although U.S. health agencies provide no accurate U.S. statistics for metabolic syndrome, we have plenty of statistics on obesity, the most common symptom of metabolic syndrome. In fact, the rising incidence of metabolic syndrome closely parallels the prevalence of obesity in America. The incidence of metabolic syndrome lags behind the incidence of obesity by about two years.

On the CDC website, you can review trends in U.S. obesity over time. The animated map on this URL shows state-by-state percentages, from 1985 to 2010, of people whose body mass index is 30 or higher: www.cdc.gov/obesity/data/index.htm.

The body mass index (BMI) reflects body weight adjusted for a person's height. Multiply your weight (lbs.) by 703 and divide by your height (in.) squared to find your BMI. If your BMI is higher than 25, you're overweight, according to CDC standards.

Obesity is more common among Hispanics and Native Americans of both sexes and more common among African American women than among European Americans. High blood pressure, diabetes, and heart disease are more prevalent in Native Americans, African Americans, and Latinos than in European Americans. Ethnicities with high skin melanin are at greater risk, and women and children are the fastest-growing sectors of these populations at risk.

New Obesity Trend Map from CDC

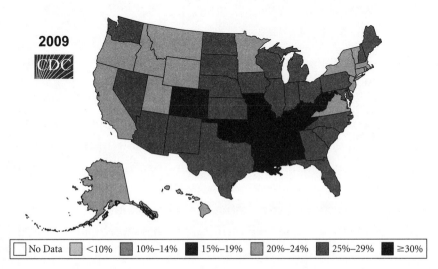

2009

| | No Data | | <10% | | 10%–14% | | 15%–19% | | 20%–24% | | 25%–29% | | ≥30% |

Annual obesity maps of U.S. populations show that Mississippi stays ahead of the rest of the country in the prevalence of obesity, and this is also the state with the highest percentage of African Americans, based on 2000 census data. Obesity was 51 percent more common in African Americans and 21 percent more common in Latin Americans than in European Americans. This suggests that vitamin D deficiency risk and obesity often go hand in hand.

Men's Health Magazine has awarded Houston, Detroit, and Philadelphia the dubious title of "Fattest Cities in America," and these three places are also among the top five cities with the most African Americans or combined African American designation (2000 census). Furthermore, African Americans in the North and the Midwest typically live in large metropolitan areas, and studies show that urban dwellers have lower vitamin D levels than residents of rural areas.

Size Matters

Population studies also reveal a significant statistic—that if you started life as a full-term infant whose weight was low at birth due to poor nutrition, you're more likely to grow up

- to become obese;
- to have type 2 diabetes; and/or
- to have high blood pressure

Epidemiological studies in the United Kingdom, the Netherlands, and India also show that low-birth-weight babies who have fast catch-up growth in early childhood are more likely than their peers to develop obesity, high blood pressure, diabetes, and/or heart disease. It's also clear that African Americans have low-birth-weight and very-low-birth-weight babies more than twice as often as European Americans.

One study showed that infants are longer, are heavier, and have lower bone-mineral content if their mothers have low vitamin D levels, even when these aren't classic examples of "nutritional deprivation."

This is consistent with the role vitamin D plays in slowing growth and promoting cell differentiation.

Other studies show us how vitamin D works. Researchers looking at Indians living in the United Kingdom saw that last-trimester vitamin D supplementation of nutrition-deficient pregnant women who were eating low-protein vegetarian diets made these women gain weight faster in the third trimester and have infants half as likely to have intrauterine growth retardation. This information suggests that vitamin D and diet play important roles in fetal development and future risk for metabolic syndrome.

If you are born with a risk for metabolic syndrome, this dicey heritage may be carried to fruition if you fail to get enough sun or physical activity and you take in too many of the taboo foods: grains, cheese, and salt.

Large-population studies in the United States and Norway tell us that people who fail to get enough vitamin D will increase their chances of having high blood pressure, obesity, and diabetes. Numerous studies also point to a greater likelihood of obesity, high blood pressure, diabetes, heart attacks, and strokes if you eat a diet low in omega-3 fatty acids and magnesium.

SHARON'S WEIGHT GAIN AND PAIN

When Sharon, forty-five, came to see me, she told me that she'd had three years of pain and stiffness in her knees, shoulders, and hands. One doctor had told her she had osteoarthritis in her knees and treated her with several nonsteroidal anti-inflammatory drugs (NSAIDs), such as ibuprofen, but since she had stopped taking them, her pain had increased. Along with the other symptoms, she'd gained 10 pounds and felt anxious and tired. She rarely slept well. She weighed 180 pounds. Except for grinding behind both kneecaps, her joints were normal, although her bones and muscles were tender. Sharon's overall health was normal.

On her first visit to our offices, Sharon had scores of 0.625–65–75–55–4 (function, pain, fatigue, health perception, sleep).

In the morning, she had about ten minutes of stiffness. Lab studies were normal; her vitamin D level was 29, PTH was 51, and calcium was normal. She started taking vitamin D and began avoiding salt, cheese, and grains. She changed her diet to a 3:1 ratio of fresh produce to lean meat.

The changes made a big difference in her scores when we saw her three months later. She posted 0.625–40–40–40–5, and reported five minutes per day of stiffness. She'd lost weight, too—Sharon now weighed 167 pounds. Her vitamin D level was 32. But we saw an unexpected increase in her PTH, which was 73; this pointed to protein and/or magnesium deficiency, which often accompanies vitamin D deficiency. So she boosted her protein intake and began supplementing her magnesium, too.

After six months on the Vitamin D Cure, she had scores of 0.5–30–35–40–7 and only five minutes of morning stiffness. Her weight was down to 158 and her vitamin D level rose to 54.

This shows how much weight a person can lose via vitamin D normalization and dietary modification. Sharon lost 22 pounds in six months, and she wasn't even on a diet!

The beneficial effects of vitamin D and a good diet on fatigue, pain, and weight in just six months were amazing. She saw a 50 percent reduction in her pain and fatigue, and her sleep quality improved.

What's great is that the Vitamin D Cure doesn't just suppress symptoms, it also addresses the cause of the symptoms.

To Feel Full, Eat Protein

The feeling of satisfaction and fullness after a meal comes from several signals, including your stomach's degree of distention and the foods you ate. Animal and human studies show that protein is the nutrient most likely to make you feel full. When rodents are given the choice of a diet high in carbohydrate, protein, or fat, they will choose a high-protein meal.

In 2004, Drs. Thomas Halton and Frank Hu of the Harvard University School of Public Health compared the satiety factor of high-protein diets to high-carbohydrate and low-fat diets, and they concluded that you feel more satisfied if you follow a high-protein diet, which, in turn, will result in your consuming fewer calories. This makes you lose more weight—and sustain the loss—than you would if you have a high-carb or a low-fat diet.

The basics to take away from these studies of weight-loss programs are two simple facts:

1. To lose weight, you have to be able to stay on the program.

2. To stay on the program, you have to feel satisfied on the program.

Calcium is also linked to satiety, and people who take in a great deal of calcium often have a lower body mass index. When they increase their calcium intake and restrict calories, people lose more weight than they do without calcium supplementation, but this may occur only because they are making up for lack of vitamin D.

Dr. Wendy Chan She Ping-Delfos of Curtin University in Australia looked at what people ate for twenty-four hours following two kinds of breakfasts. One was low in calcium and low in vitamin D. The other was high in calcium and high in vitamin D.

People who ate the high-calcium, high-D breakfast consumed an average of three hundred fewer calories in the twenty-four hours following breakfast. This supports the belief that you feel fuller and more satisfied if you start your day with a breakfast high in vitamin D and calcium.

Looking for Nutrition in All the Wrong Places

Your appetite craves specific nutrients, not calories. That means the trick is making sure you consume the nutrients your body craves so you can satisfy your hunger and stop eating sooner. This is a great way to control your weight!

In the United States, a person typically consumes 3,300 milligrams of dietary sodium per day, according to the National Health and Nutrition

Examination Survey database. This is 40 percent *more than* you should have.

An American's average intake of potassium is about 2,600 milligrams a day, but you need 4,700 milligrams a day, according to the National Academy of Sciences. The average intake of magnesium is 270 milligrams a day, but the recommended amount is 400 milligrams a day.

Perhaps this is the real story behind your cravings:

- You crave chocolate because it's high in magnesium and you're deficient in magnesium.

- You crave cheese because you're calcium-deficient due to vitamin D deficiency.

- You crave grain because this is a convenient protein and you're conditioned to the sweetness—but it's *not* a good source of protein.

Many of us respond to the cries of hunger with the wrong choices—ones that bring along too many calories and too little nutrition. Instead, we should be answering our hunger pangs with lean meat, green vegetables, fruit, and nuts. These will satisfy you in smaller caloric packages simply because they provide what you need more efficiently *and* specifically. Keep those foods handy!

This plan works so well that many people eliminate the need for blood pressure medications, lose weight, and experience other amazing health improvements.

Stop Your Soaring Blood Pressure

We know that your blood pressure can soar for many reasons. Big factors are kidney function and the relationship between your kidneys and the adrenal glands on top of your kidneys. For normal blood pressure, you need a proper balance of hormones. Your adrenal glands and kidneys produce blood pressure–spiking substances— cortisol, adrenaline, renin, angiotensin, and aldosterone. Renin, angiotensin, and aldosterone raise blood pressure in adults, but a fetus needs an appropriate balance of these hormones for normal kidney development.

Mice with nonfunctioning vitamin D systems develop high blood pressure and enlarged hearts. This has been tied to increased production of renin and angiotensin from the kidney. Vitamin D suppresses the gene for renin, and without D, renin goes up and angiotensin follows, raising blood pressure.

When Dr. John Forman and his colleagues at Harvard University analyzed data from the Health Professionals Follow-Up Study and Nurses Health Study groups, they found that during four years of follow-up, a vitamin D level lower than 15 ng/mL increased the risk of high blood pressure more than sixfold in men and nearly threefold in women when compared to those whose vitamin D levels were at or above 30 ng/mL.

Dr. Stephen Rostand of the University of Alabama has shown that the farther you live from the equator, the greater your chances of having high blood pressure. This is true worldwide. When people with high skin melanin migrate from the equator, they often develop high blood pressure.

Dr. Michael Holick at Boston University confirmed the connection between UVB light and high blood pressure. When people with high blood pressure were exposed to enough UVB light to produce a 162 percent rise in vitamin D levels, their blood pressure dropped (both upper and lower numbers—systolic and diastolic). This didn't happen in the study participants who were exposed to UVA light only. What led to a drop in blood pressure was the vitamin D production UVB light had facilitated.

Vitamin D supplementation works about the same way. When Dr. Michael Pfeifer at the Gustav Pommer Institute in Hamburg, Germany, gave 148 elderly women 1,200 milligrams of calcium a day, with or without 800 IU of vitamin D per day, those in the vitamin D supplementation group had a 72 percent increase in D levels, a 9.3 percent reduction in systolic blood pressure, and a slowing of the heart rate by 5.4 percent. Twice as many in the vitamin D group had a 5-millimeter drop in systolic pressure compared to the calcium-only group.

Vitamin D and Diabetes

With type 1 diabetes, an autoimmune disease, early in childhood development your immune system begins to make antibodies to islet cells that manufacture insulin in the pancreas. These antibodies destroy the islet cells, and the production of insulin declines, producing diabetes symptoms.

Type 2 diabetes is characterized by impairment in insulin release as well as insulin resistance in muscles, fat cells, and the liver. Insulin resistance often accompanies aging and obesity, and dietary factors and inactivity make it worse.

You need extra insulin to overcome insulin resistance. The high insulin levels of type 2 diabetes contribute to diabetes complications, including cholesterol abnormalities, diabetic eye disease, diabetic kidney disease, and vascular disease.

Type 2 diabetes is like a car trying to pull a trailer that's too large. The car overheats, isn't fuel efficient, and wears out faster. You would trade your car in for a truck that has towing capacity, but the problem is, you can't just go out and buy a larger pancreas to handle your diabetes.

In animal studies, Dr. Anthony Norman of the University of California at Riverside showed that vitamin D is necessary for the pancreas to release insulin. Vitamin D deficiency produces insulin resistance in tissues.

Right in line with these animal studies are results of the Third National Health and Nutrition Examination Survey and the Women's Health Study Data, which showed that low vitamin D and calcium intake led to metabolic syndrome. In the Women's Health Study, the relationship was stronger with calcium than vitamin D; in the National Health and Nutrition Examination Survey III, both low vitamin D and calcium were independently associated with higher risk for developing metabolic syndrome.

In 2009, researchers at Massey University in Auckland, New Zealand, gave forty-two insulin-resistant South Asian women 4,000 IU of vitamin D$_3$ daily for six months. These subjects showed a significant improvement in insulin sensitivity and insulin resistance. The thirty-nine who did not receive vitamin D_3 did not improve. Scientists have seen similar results in men with dark skin tones but not in fair-skinned Europeans.

For more information on diabetes, see http://ndep.nih.gov/.

A Heart-to-Heart Moment

Another aspect of metabolic syndrome is an increased risk for heart and vascular disease, including heart attacks, strokes, peripheral vascular disease, and heart failure. Historically, researchers have linked elevated cholesterol (especially LDL), high triglycerides and low HDL with these diseases. Vitamin D deficiency has been linked to most risk factors for vascular disease, such as high triglycerides and low HDL relative to total cholesterol. Vitamin D deficiency hasn't been linked to high total cholesterol or high LDL, however.

Since the first edition of this book was published in 2008, numerous studies have shown an increased risk of heart and vascular disease in populations with vitamin D deficiency. In 2008, Dr. Thomas J. Wang and his colleagues at Harvard University published one of the first studies citing such a relationship in the journal *Circulation*. They studied about two thousand people from the Framingham Offspring Cohort and found that a vitamin D level lower than 15 ng/mL was associated with a 62 percent increase in the risk of future heart and vascular disease. If a person had high blood pressure and vitamin D deficiency, he or she had twice the risk.

Harvard University investigators reported similar findings from the Health Professionals Follow-Up Study. In this research, vitamin D levels lower than 30 ng/mL were associated with nearly twice the risk of heart attack.

You can extend the findings for cardiovascular events to death from cardiovascular disease or death from any cause. Drs. Dobnig and Pilz and their colleagues in Germany and Austria were the first to show that vitamin D deficiency was linked to higher cardiovascular mortality and all-cause mortality. Evaluation of the Third National Health and Nutrition Examination Survey in 2009 found that older Americans with severe vitamin D deficiency (<10 ng/mL) had 2.4- and 1.8-fold greater likelihood of cardiovascular and all-cause mortality, respectively, when compared with vitamin D–sufficient participants (≥40 ng/mL). The Tromsø Study population in Norway showed similar results.

Dietary surveys tell us that when people increase their intake of dark meat/coldwater fish, they have fewer heart attacks and strokes and fewer deaths from heart attacks and strokes. The improved health outcomes have always been credited to the omega-3 fats in these fish, but the same dietary sources are also high in vitamin D. (Coldwater, wild-caught, ocean-going fish usually have a dark red color to the meat, which makes it easy to spot fish that's high in omega-3.)

Vitamin D, Inflammation, and the Metabolic Syndrome

Our understanding of cardiovascular disease has recently shifted from a simple focus on lipids to a focus on inflammation. The weight of evidence now suggests that chronic low-grade inflammation and its effect on blood vessels are actually what cause arteriosclerosis (coronary heart disease). Furthermore, diet and fat cells are the sources of this inflammation, and clear links between inflammation and low vitamin D levels have been shown.

Saturated fat from foods such as cheese and processed meats increase the production of inflammatory substances. Fat cells are biologically active; they don't just store energy, they produce hormones and molecules that affect metabolism and promote inflammation. Vitamin D may counteract this inflammation. When inflammatory cells stick to the walls of blood vessels and are activated, they cause blood vessel damage that leads to plaque formation (arteriosclerosis); but vitamin D reduces the stickiness of the blood vessel-lining cells and calms white blood cells that might otherwise become inflamed.

A study published in the *American Journal of Hypertension* in 2011 looked at fortification of vitamin D and its effects on blood vessel function. Researchers found that correcting vitamin D deficiency during a sixteen-week period enhanced the dilation of blood vessels in response to blood flow and reduced stress on the walls of the blood vessels. Study subjects were African Americans, who are at higher risk for both vitamin D deficiency and high blood pressure.

Those in the study who didn't receive vitamin D showed no improvements in these measures. The decreased stress on the blood vessels may account for the lower risk of heart attacks and strokes in patients with higher vitamin D levels.

Diet and the Metabolic Syndrome

Normalizing vitamin D alone will not prevent development of the metabolic syndrome because you have to improve your diet, too. But increased intake of lean protein, vitamin D, and fresh produce will make you less hungry, so you'll eat fewer calories automatically.

It's as simple as this: eating lots of veggies packed with potassium and magnesium will make you feel fuller. But to accomplish this, you'll have to cut down on cheese and grain, which aren't nutrient-dense. Make these changes in your eating and you'll have fewer troubles with your weight, blood pressure, diabetes, and cholesterol.

Interpreting the DASH Diet

DASH (Dietary Approaches to Stop High Blood Pressure) looked at the relationship between blood pressure and Americans' intake of potassium, magnesium, and calcium. This study, published in the *New England Journal of Medicine* in 1997, investigated the diets of minorities (mostly African Americans) who had modest high blood pressure and ones who didn't have high blood pressure. The participants followed three different diets for eight weeks each, and researchers monitored their blood pressure.

The control diet was low in potassium, magnesium, and calcium. The second diet was high in fruits and vegetables and rich in potassium and magnesium but low in calcium due to the absence of dairy. The third—a combination diet—added low-fat dairy to the fruit-and-vegetable diet and reduced the saturated fat. All of the diets provided the same amount of calories and salt.

African Americans with high blood pressure and those without high blood pressure all lowered their blood pressure numbers, and those with high blood pressure on the combination diet showed the greatest reduction. The blood pressure reduction in this group, amazingly, mirrored that of people who take blood pressure medication.

The DASH diet also had beneficial effects on other aspects of the metabolic syndrome. The combination diet caused a 50 percent improvement in insulin sensitivity.

In a separate study looking at the effect the DASH diet had on metabolic syndrome symptoms in Iranian men and women, Dr. Leila Azadbakht saw reduced waist circumferences and body weight. In fact, the DASH diet worked better than a calorie-restricted diet. Compared to the calorie-restricted diet, the DASH diet also significantly lowered triglycerides and raised HDL, and it lowered fasting blood sugar more efficiently.

A diet high in potassium, magnesium, and calcium reduces body weight, improves body proportions, lowers blood pressure, corrects lipid abnormalities, and improves insulin sensitivity. Furthermore, people stick with this healthy diet to the tune of about 95 percent of participants because they aren't forced to sacrifice taste or satisfaction.

The Mediterranean Difference

The Mediterranean diet emphasizes healthy fat intake. You get monounsaturated fat from olive oil and omega-3 fatty acids from dark-meat fish; you increase your vegetable and fruit intake; and you eat fewer refined carbs. Metabolic syndrome sufferers who stayed on this diet for two years had greater reductions than control-diet participants in these areas:

- Weight
- Waist circumference
- Blood pressure
- Total cholesterol
- Triglycerides
- Fasting glucose
- Insulin

They had greater increases in their HDL levels as well.

Study directors Dr. Katherine Esposito and her colleagues at the University of Naples in Italy also measured the levels of inflammatory substances associated with heart attacks and strokes and found that the study participants on the Mediterranean diet had lower levels of all inflammatory substances than those on the control diet. These same people also showed greatly improved blood vessel wall function, with dilation of blood vessels and decreased platelet sticking.

Clearly, omega-3 fatty acids and monounsaturated fats, along with increased intake of vegetables and fruits, are important to your health. To reverse the havoc the metabolic syndrome wreaks, you simply have to neutralize your acid-base imbalance.

You can accomplish this with the Vitamin D Cure eating plan, which, like the DASH diet and the Mediterranean diet, asks you to eat more vegetables and fruits (these provide large amounts of antacid). With these diets, you also take in greater amounts of omega-3 fatty acids compared to omega-6 fats and saturated fats, so these things all synch up to produce excellent health benefits.

Going Paleolithic

The big advantage of the Vitamin D Cure eating plan is that it takes the DASH and Mediterranean diets one step farther. Here's how the idea evolved.

Three-fourths of people worldwide are lactose-intolerant, which means they don't digest dairy products well. And at least half of the world's population is vitamin D deficient due to lack of sun exposure and bad diet/malnutrition. Grain, although inexpensive, is a poor source of protein, omega-3 fats, magnesium, calcium, potassium, and vitamins, and it generates an inordinate amount of acid in the American diet. About 1 percent or more of the world's population is allergic to gluten—a protein in wheat, barley, rye, and (sometimes) oats, causing bowel inflammation that leads to faulty absorption and vitamin D deficiency.

We know that you're better off eating more lean protein and three times as much produce as protein. This raises a question: why not eliminate dairy and grains from the DASH and Mediterranean diets and replace them with vitamin D, more lean meat (especially dark-meat fish), and more green produce? After all, this is what our Paleolithic/Stone Age ancestors ate and what we were designed to eat.

It's easy to correct your calcium imbalance by normalizing your vitamin D levels with sun and supplements, and you can avoid the problem of lactose intolerance by eliminating dairy. If you neutralize the acid in your diet by consuming three times as much produce as lean protein, you reduce your calcium requirements and ensure adequate magnesium and potassium intake along with the associated antacids. By avoiding grains, you avoid gluten allergies and a lot of extra calories. In addition, green, leafy vegetables have more fiber and nutrients—keys to good health—than even fortified grain can give you. Finally, restoring a healthy ratio of omega-6 to omega-3 fat (less than or equal to 5:1) reduces inflammation and its damage to blood vessels.

Moving Out of the Metabolic Syndrome

Exercise, vitamin D supplementation, and a good diet can keep you from becoming obese, no matter what your gene pool. Exercise makes vitamin D work for you via metabolism changes and increased sun exposure; it directs the flow of nutrients into bone and muscle rather than fat (see chapter 8).

Exercise also triggers the production of endorphins (a morphinelike substance) in the brain, reducing your desire for certain foods. When you exercise, you produce more serotonin and other hormones that curb appetite. Cardio exercise does you many favors. It

- reduces depression;
- improves sleep;
- burns calories;
- liberates vitamin D;
- lowers inflammation;
- improves insulin sensitivity; and
- reduces your risk of cardiovascular disease, diabetes, and dementia.

You get so much bang for your buck out of cardio that it's something you definitely want to include in your week's activities.

Lowering Your Risk

The recommendations in the Vitamin D Cure are estimated to lower your risk of obesity by 57 percent, lower your risk of high blood pressure by 67 percent, and lower your risk of glucose intolerance by 55 percent. These changes also translate into a 50 percent lower risk of heart attacks and strokes.

10

The Vitamin D Cure
for Mood and Memory

Vitamin D goes to work at the moment of conception and doesn't quit until someone's writing your epitaph. The fact is, if you have enough D and combine it with a healthy diet and exercise, you'll probably have a sharp mind when you're in your nineties and beyond.

Vitamin D has a great deal to do with how well your brain works throughout your life. It's extremely important because D is essential to proper brain function.

Consider the roles that vitamin D plays in brain work. Vitamin D

- controls brain development in the fetus through a sculpting process that turns off or eliminates certain nerve cells while allowing others to grow;

- facilitates learning by stimulating nerve growth factors;

- serves as an antioxidant in the adult brain and protects it from injury;

- suppresses key mediators of inflammation (nuclear factors cytokines, prostaglandins) and;

- regulates the repair process when there's damage, using some of the same growth factors required for brain development.

At the same time, you also need good food choices to get the most out of your brain. Diet and D are great partners. They have a strong alliance because a healthy diet enhances vitamin D's ability to take care of its jobs. By the same token, though, a bad diet can hinder vitamin D in its efforts. And many people who are eating a bad diet don't realize that their food choices are counterproductive to good health.

Here's how your diet fosters brain growth:

- Your brain needs protein and polyunsaturated fats (especially DHA) to grow correctly. These are critical building blocks.

- DHA works with vitamin D to direct the sculpting process and promote your ability to learn.

- Dietary acid-base balance can affect favorably or unfavorably the levels of hormones in the brain that work alone and together with vitamin D to direct brain development and brain function.

- Cheese and refined grains promote inflammation that may overwhelm brain protective mechanisms, causing degenerative neurological disease. Conversely, fresh green produce and lean meat that's high in omega-3 fats suppress inflammation and protect brain function.

Here's how a lack of vitamin D leads to development of certain diseases.

Malnutrition during fetal development increases the risk of a person's developing diabetes and heart disease later in life (see chapter 9). This early programming is then amplified by poor diet and lack of exercise to produce insulin resistance and chronic low-grade inflammation, which may lead to disease.

It now appears that schizophrenia, depression, dementia, and other psychological diseases, including chronic pain, may result from similar early programming (malnutrition, infection, emotional trauma) amplified by chronic low-grade brain inflammation. An environment or a family situation that is not emotionally nurturing, nutritional deficiencies, and lack of mental and physical exercise contribute to the chronic low-grade brain inflammation.

This puts the Vitamin D Cure lifestyle front and center. Now the anti-inflammatory and antioxidant effects of vitamin D and omega-3 fats become important in reducing brain inflammation and its effects on mood, memory, and pain. The Vitamin D Cure diet complements these effects by eliminating ingredients that promote inflammation and adding foods that enhance, repair, and establish new nerve connections. Adding exercise and meditation to your lifestyle further calms the inflammation, elevates mood, and enhances your brain's ability to learn and remember.

Developing Brain Disorders

Scientists have categorized disorders of the developing brain to include autism, schizophrenia, attention deficit hyperactivity disorder (ADHD), and bipolar disorder. Evidence shows that early emotional and biological stressors, such as infections and nutritional deficiencies, combine with genetic risk to alter brain structure and brain function, from mood to memory to more complex behaviors such as socialization.

Dr. John J. McGrath and his colleagues at Griffith University in Brisbane, Queensland, Australia, found that vitamin D deficiency during fetal development in rodents altered the expression of dozens of the offspring's genes, including nerve growth factors and structural proteins. These variations in gene and protein expression changed the size and shape of the brain, with cells replicating more frequently than normal. These brain changes were accompanied by a variety of complex behavioral changes that persisted into the adult years of these animals.

Vitamin D deficiency (see chapter 11) has broad effects on the immune system that increase the overall production of inflammatory substances and activate inflammatory cells inappropriately. Plus, vitamin D deficiency appears to impair the ability of the immune system to fight infection, which is important in pregnancy and early childhood—when the brain is developing and vulnerable.

The complex disease schizophrenia is marked by bizarre delusions (psychosis), social withdrawal, disordered memory and thinking, and extreme mood swings. This disease is usually progressive, leading to a chronic mentally debilitated state.

Risk for schizophrenia increases when a baby has an infection during infancy, has a low birth weight, or is premature; when a woman has an infection during pregnancy or preeclampsia (a complication of late pregnancy); or when someone lives in a location far from the equator. Vitamin D deficiency is associated with each of these risk factors.

Nutritional deficiencies and their consequences may increase your genetic risk. The bottom line is that you can't change your genes, but you can definitely change what you eat.

In the Finland Birth Cohort of 1966, boys who took cod liver oil, which is high in vitamins A and D and omega-3 fats, during the first year of life were much less likely to develop schizophrenia than were boys who did not take cod liver oil.

Autism is a complex disorder of brain development that affects language, socialization, cognition, and mood. Evidence suggests that autism shares a genetic risk with schizophrenia and ADHD. Similar findings—prenatal stressors, winter-spring birth, and possibly a higher risk in dark-skinned immigrants—suggest a possible connection between autism and vitamin D deficiency.

Fetal development and early childhood are vulnerable periods when vitamin D, omega-3 fats, and adequate protein and vegetables have the potential to build a brain foundation that is strong but flexible. Their absence, though, creates a shaky foundation that is more susceptible to stress and infection and may give the child a reduced ability to learn new skills, behaviors, and responses.

Vitamin D, Diet, and Chronic Pain

Chronic pain affects 15 percent of adults in the United States—about 45 million people. The most common single location of chronic pain is in the lower back, but as many as 60 percent of these people hurt in many places.

The most common cause of such pain is arthritis and bone diseases. CDC research shows that people with arthritis and chronic pain have a higher incidence of obesity, high blood pressure, heart disease, diabetes, and smoking.

This suggests that there may be common links to all these diseases. Research suggests that those common links are vitamin D deficiency and dietary imbalance.

Today many patients with pain in multiple locations are diagnosed with fibromyalgia. Fibromyalgia (FMS) is likely an affective disorder, belonging to a family of diseases referred to by Harvard psychiatrists as affective spectrum disorder (ASD). This family of disorders also includes depression, posttraumatic stress disorder, anxiety disorders, chronic fatigue, and substance abuse syndromes. In many of these patients, some psychological trauma early in life (typically before age thirty) is the root cause of ASD.

ASD is associated with a common set of symptoms and several common biochemical features such as mood disturbance, sleep disturbance, fatigue, and musculoskeletal pain. These people's brain chemistry shows chronic activation of the hypothalamic pituitary axis (HPA).

The HPA is the brain's hormone regulatory center, which controls your stress response. An acute stress response (pounding heart, sweaty palms) occurs when the police pull you over for running a red light. That's short-term, but fibromyalgia and acid excess create chronic stress responses; they're only a fraction of the potency, but they're happening 24/7, year round. This chronic stress response leads to higher cortisol levels, lower growth hormone levels, elevated inflammation and pain-causing substance levels, and blunting of the serotonin system. In other words, your serotonin production is reduced, and doesn't respond to normal signals to increase or decrease.

Many symptoms of fibromyalgia may be worsened by vitamin D deficiency, inadequate omega-3 fats, and dietary acidosis. In fact, vitamin D and diet deficiencies are present in more than half of patients with fibromyalgia that I see in my practice. Addressing these deficiencies would help most people who have fibromyalgia.

We know that serotonin metabolism rises and falls with sun exposure and vitamin D production and that correcting vitamin D levels improves mood and fatigue in seasonal affective disorder.

Vitamin D deficiency increases the production of the kidney hormone renin, which can make you release more stress hormones. Lack of vitamin D is associated with higher levels of inflammatory substances in the blood and brain. This inflammation triggers a chronic stress response, producing insomnia and chronic fatigue, which amplify pain. Dietary acidosis increases the production of cortisol, and other forms of acidosis are associated with high prolactin levels, both of which are often abnormalities of fibromyalgia.

Magnesium deficiency, which results from inadequate intake and an acidic diet, can give you a lower pain threshold. We know that giving supplemental magnesium to patients before surgery can lower the amount of anesthesia required and reduce the need for postoperative pain medication.

Migraine headaches, common in people with fibromyalgia, respond well to magnesium supplementation. In several placebo-controlled trials, researchers gave patients magnesium sulfate intravenously, and this eliminated the aura and nausea associated with migraines and reduced head pain partially or completely in 40 to 85 percent of patients. In more than half, relief lasted 24 hours or more.

ANSELLA'S FIBROMYALGIA

Ansella, sixty-two, had been diagnosed with chronic fatigue syndrome and fibromyalgia when she first came to see me seven years ago. She also had moderate to severe osteoarthritis in her knees and suffered from headaches and irritable bowel syndrome. Ansella was taking antidepressants and narcotics for symptom control, and she wanted me to prescribe guaifenesin, even though she had been taking this supplement for several years with no measurable improvements.

I asked her if we could add a new dimension to her regimen. I measured her vitamin D level, evaluated her diet, and found that she had a very low vitamin D level—only 24 nanograms per milliliter in the month of June.

She began vitamin D replacement and made dietary changes, and when she filled out our CLINHAQII questionnaire a year later, her scores were 1.625–20–60–20–5, even though she was taking much less medication. Her pain had dropped by 75 percent; she no longer had headaches; and she was less tired. Ansella felt worlds better.

When chronic pain is all over the body, doctors often label it fibromyalgia. Yet some of these people are suffering from severe vitamin D deficiency, or osteomalacia. They have migratory pain that waxes and wanes—referred to as their "good days and bad days." When the pain is severe, they hurt around the clock. In most cases, pain medications don't help much.

A study at the Mayo Clinic in Minnesota looked at vitamin D levels in people who hurt all over (muscles and bones) but had no diagnosis that explained the cause of the pain. More than 90 percent had D levels below 20; 28 percent had levels of 8 or less. (A normal vitamin D level is at least 35.) Participants were African Americans, East Africans, Hispanics, and Native Americans.

Those who took vitamin D supplements saw dramatic resolution of pain, fatigue, and muscle cramps. Study author Dr. Gregory Plotnikoff, from the University of Minnesota Center for Spirituality and Healing, found that these people's severe vitamin D deficiency was what had caused increased bone remodeling and subsequent skeletal pain. Normalizing their vitamin D and calcium metabolism fixed the problems: no more pain, no more fatigue, no more muscle cramps.

Researchers saw similar improvements in a study at Riyadh Armed Forces Hospital in Saudi Arabia. The vitamin D levels of 360 people with chronic back pain for more than six months were tested, and 83 percent had vitamin D deficiency. Then, when doctors normalized their D levels, back pain improved in all of them. Two-thirds of those who'd had normal D levels also saw improvements in their back pain with supplementation.

Blue Moods

I met Roseanna in 2004 when she accompanied her mother on an office visit because she had questions about the supplements and diet I'd prescribed for her mother. Although her mother was feeling much better (three months earlier, she'd complained of extreme fatigue and severe generalized pain), Roseanna was skeptical about the high doses of vitamin D and the dietary modifications.

As I explained the prevalence of vitamin D deficiency and dietary acid-base imbalance and listed the risk factors for developing D deficiency, Roseanna told me that she and her husband, Kyle, both suffered from depression that was much worse in the winter. Apparently her husband had severe symptoms, and his health had declined even more since they retired and moved to Anchorage, Alaska, at 61 degrees north latitude. Of course, my jaw dropped when she said "Alaska." Not enough sun, not enough vitamin D!

Next, Roseanna and her husband came to see me when they were visiting for the holidays. Both Roseanna and Kyle had severe vitamin D deficiency; their levels were 18, and their PTH levels were elevated. Fortunately, they began vitamin D supplementation and were able to eliminate their seasonal depression, year-round fatigue, and muscle aches.

I've seen numerous people who have seasonal affective disorder (SAD), which the U.S. Department of Health and Human Services defines in the following way: "Seasonal Depression, also known as Seasonal Affective Disorder (SAD), can occur among individuals with major or minor depression. An essential feature of this condition is the onset and remission of depressive episodes at certain times of the year. In most cases, episodes start in the fall or winter and stop in the spring. Recurrent depressive episodes may also occur in the summer but less frequently."

Seasonal affective disorder can even have lethal extremes. Dr. Gavin Lambert of Baker Medical Research Institute in Australia found that suicide rates peak in the spring just after winter's end. This seasonal variation also showed up in other studies.

At the same time, this phenomenon was absent when we reviewed suicide rates in an equatorial population in Singapore. This suggests that it takes a shorter summer with UVB rays and a longer winter without UVB rays and decreased vitamin D production for the seasonal suicide trend to occur.

In fact, study participants who had traditional broad-spectrum light therapy raised their vitamin D levels only by half as much and didn't reduce their depression at all. So vitamin D replacement is more effective than light therapy for the treatment of seasonal affective disorder.

Recent research has focused on the role that brain inflammation plays in driving anhedonia (the inability to experience pleasure), loss of motivation, and depression. Observations of patients with chronic hepatitis C who were treated with the inflammatory substance interferon universally report depressed mood, disturbed sleep, lack of motivation, and even suicidal thoughts. Conversely, rheumatoid arthritis patients who were treated with antibodies that block the inflammatory substance tumor necrosis factor (TNF) reported an elevated mood and sense of well-being.

The transcription factor, NF-κB, regulates the DNA expression of inflammatory signals (IL-1, IL-6, interferon, and TNF among others) from immune system cells. Once inflammatory signals cross the blood-brain interface, they can influence the synthesis, release, and reuptake of mood-relevant neurotransmitters, including serotonin, norepinephrine, and dopamine. This transcription factor is found in different cell types throughout the brain as well as the immune system. Vitamin D is known to inactivate NF-κB blocking production of a number of inflammatory substances both in the blood and the brain. This mechanism probably accounts for some of its mood-enhancing properties.

Historically, serotonin has been at the center of most discussions about the brain chemistry of depression until recent research on inflammation and brain function superseded it. But don't count serotonin out. The amino acid tryptophan can be converted into serotonin and melatonin or into kynurenic acid and quinolinic acid in the brain. Inflammation in the gut or in the brain favors production of the latter two neurotransmitters, which are associated with anxiety and depressed mood.

Animal studies show that exposure to vitamin D early in life influences the production and metabolism of neurotransmitters such as serotonin, dopamine, and norepinephrine, all of which are key brain substances involved in the symptoms of depression, anxiety, and addiction. The changes in the production and breakdown of these substances caused by a single exposure to vitamin D at birth persisted for two generations of animals. It is unclear how this "epigenetic effect" may influence the risk of mood disorders in humans and within families, but it will be important in determining the risk of depression and anxiety.

We also see evidence that women and men with a history of depression have lower bone mass and more signs of bone turnover, both of which are associated with vitamin D deficiency, lack of omega-3 fatty acids, and dietary acid-base imbalance.

Vitamin D, Diet, Learning, and Memory

Memory and learning are different sides of the same coin, and both are linked to brain development and the ability to make new connections between nerve cells. During brain development, your body selectively turns off nerve cells to create a sensory or motor response, like carving away excess wood or chipping away excess stone to create a sculpture. When development is complete, you have a predictable motor or sensory function, such as walking or being able to recognize the taste of a specific food.

Vitamin D and nutrients such as omega-3 fatty acids and magnesium, which are important in regulating gene expression, control this sculpting process. They select the cells that will remain to perform specific functions. Science is learning that this selection process early in life is critical in determining the quality and stability of brain structure and function and therefore learning and memory later in life. Vitamin D and nutrition direct the finished product throughout life, determining how well it performs.

Recent studies show that supplementation of omega-3 fats, especially DHA, during pregnancy improves cognitive performance of a child when he or she is four years old. Additional studies suggest that higher omega-3 fat intake preserves cognitive function as we age, reducing the risk of dementia. It's clear that omega-3 fats are important throughout life for optimal brain development and performance.

Nerve growth factors determine your brain's learning or memory capacity or its interconnectedness. We know from the results of animal studies that vitamin D controls some of these nerve growth factors and other elements that help to establish new connections and create memories. In response to brain injury, these same factors are important in repair.

Over the years, your brain accumulates memories and injuries. Brain injuries include emotional traumas, head traumas, damage from high blood pressure, and damage from the ravages of unhealthy living. In this situation, the brain's capacity to protect and repair cannot keep up with all of these stresses and you begin to lose brain function. This is called dementia.

Alzheimer's disease is a deterioration of understanding, memory, and processing memories for problem solving. About 10 percent of people older than sixty-five and half of those eighty-five and older develop symptoms of Alzheimer's disease, and it is more common in older people who also have obesity, hypertension, heart disease, or diabetes. Research shows that vitamin D, omega-3 fats, and magnesium can reduce the levels of inflammatory substances that nerve cells produce following brain injury, thereby limiting damage.

Recent data from the NAME (Nutrition, Aging, and Memory in Elders) study, analyzed at Tufts University, reveals consistent connections between low vitamin D levels and poor cognitive performance. Brain imaging suggests that this increased risk is due to vascular disease within the brain (see chapter 9). Alzheimer's research at Washington University in St. Louis found that 58 percent of eighty patients had vitamin D levels of 20 or lower. Participants' mood disturbances, depression, and understanding were studied, and those with vitamin D levels below 20 were eleven times more likely to have a mood disorder and three times more likely to have impaired understanding. People with Alzheimer's disease who have early comprehension troubles that progress to dementia quickly usually have very low vitamin D levels. Experts believe that low D levels probably play a role in the progression of dementia.

A person in the late stages of Parkinson's disease also may have dementia that's much like that seen in Alzheimer's disease. The dysfunctional movements of Parkinson's disease point to the source of the problem in an area at the base of the brain that coordinates movement. This region of the brain has a very high concentration of vitamin D receptors. Specialized cells in this area produce the neurotransmitter dopamine. Deterioration of these cells in Parkinson's disease reduces the production of dopamine, which leads to the loss of coordinated movement. Intriguingly, dopamine can actually bind to the vitamin D receptor.

In short, current evidence suggests that a lack of vitamin D, dietary magnesium, and omega-3 fatty acids makes it more likely that you'll have degenerative brain disease and that it will progress.

So, increase your vitamin D for a better brain!

Lowering Your Risk

The recommendations in the Vitamin D Cure are expected to almost eliminate seasonal affective disorder. A growing amount of information also suggests that fortification of vitamin D and diet combined with exercise will substantially lower your risk of depression and chronic pain, especially pain due to bone and joint disease. If implemented during fetal development and through early childhood, the Vitamin D Cure is likely to reduce the risk of schizophrenia, Parkinson's disease, and dementia.

11

The Vitamin D Cure to Optimize Your Immune System

When you're born, assuming things go well, your immune system will soak up the information it needs to do its three main jobs:

1. Recognize self from non-self (tolerance)
2. Protect against pathological infection from viruses, bacteria, and fungi
3. Repair or remove damaged or abnormal cells

But even though your immune system is hardwired for these functions, logical questions arise:

- How does your immune system distinguish bacteria-induced food poisoning from normal intestinal bacteria and sinusitis from normal nose bacteria?

- Does your immune system get a crash course in knowing when something needs repair or what the maintenance schedule is?

- Exactly how can your immune system tell the good guys (normal cells) from the bad guys (cancer cells)?

The beauty of the immune system is its ability to differentiate between what is you inherently and what isn't you and poses a threat. That is the basic lesson your immune system must learn early in life—what doesn't belong and what is friend or foe.

During fetal development, your immune system was exposed to all of the proteins in your body as your organs developed. This occurred in the protected environment of the placenta, where both fetal and maternal immune systems were suppressed. After you were born, this protected environment continued during breastfeeding, when you were exposed to foods, environmental dust and pollen, bacteria, viruses, and fungi. Breast milk contained antibodies from your mother that provided continued protection while you were being introduced to a new environment. At this time in your development, vitamin D was crucial in regulating your immune system and your mother's.

After you, as a baby, stopped breastfeeding, you caught every cold and virus that came your way during preschool, which gave your immune system an education for a lifetime. Vaccinations also "schooled" your immune system and helped you avoid life-threatening infections. Vitamin D was in the mix, too, helping to limit the frequency and severity of infections while your immune system was still learning the necessary information.

As years passed, the memory of these exposures that occurred while you were protected by your mother's antibodies and afterwards during childhood helped define your immune system's defense capabilities. Later in life, these key memories played an essential part in recognizing cells that were damaged, infected, or abnormal, such as cancer cells—and vitamin D helped form and file these memories for later use.

The Immune System Team

The immune system has two forms of protection—nonspecific protection (innate) and specific protection (adaptive).

Nonspecific Protection

The innate immune system provides nonspecific protection against invaders and threats. Our skin, mucous membranes, and the fluids produced from our lungs, stomach, eyes, mouth, and joints all provide nonspecific protection against infection, along with giving nutrients to these membranes. The integrity or toughness of these membranes is dependent on vitamin D, and vitamin D is actually found in these fluids.

The cells in these membranes can produce pathogen recognition proteins (PRP)—small cell surface receptors that recognize bacteria or virus coat proteins. Toll-like receptors are an example of a diverse family of these receptors. The numbers of toll-like receptors increase when there is plenty of vitamin D. When bacteria activate these receptors, this promotes the production of the active form of vitamin D. Activated vitamin D then triggers the production of antimicrobial proteins (defensin, cathelacidin), which kill the invading organism.

A variety of immune system cells (white blood cells) are also part of the nonspecific response. Here, the focus is on only three of these special white blood cells: macrophages (M-cells), dendritic cells (D-cells), and natural killer T (NKT) cells. Dendritic cells and NKT cells are essential bridges that link the nonspecific protection to the specific immune response when targeting an invader. All of these cell types can produce and respond to activated vitamin D.

Macrophages or M-cells are scavengers that rummage through the garbage that phagocytic cells and other cells leave behind as they search for clues to problems. They are like public watchdogs, and they present pieces of evidence to T-cells to initiate the specific immune response.

Dendritic cells are specialized M-cells. Think of them as detectives that are key to the development of tolerance to you and your friendly environment. D-cells are in your bone marrow and the lymph tissue of your spleen, tonsils, lymph nodes, lungs, and intestines, where your body often comes in contact with foreign proteins, viruses, bacteria, and fungi. D-cells have numerous vitamin D receptors, and vitamin D plays a fundamental role in restraining or suppressing the activation of D-cells early in immune system development to enable tolerance. Failure to tolerate your own proteins or good bacteria, due in part to vitamin D deficiency, may lead to autoimmune disease.

NKT cells are natural killer cells that share some features of T-cells. These cells appear to react primarily to proteins on the surface of viruses and bacteria. Invariant or iNKT cells appear to be very important for establishing and remembering tolerance to your body and your friendly bacteria. Vitamin D determines how many iNKT cells evolve from the thymus (the lymph gland that makes T-cells) in the developing immune system (fetal and early childhood). Lack of iNKT cells is found in most humans with autoimmune diseases and most animal models of human autoimmune diseases. Restoration of NKT cell numbers in animal models suppresses autoimmune disease activity. Vitamin D deficiency during fetal development or early childhood reduces iNKT cell numbers, increasing the risk for autoimmunity.

Specific Protection

The adaptive immune response is specific and reproducible (memory). This is the protection your body acquires via vaccinations and previous infections. Adaptive immune response is a specific response that can be recalled for protection in the future. Skin offers nonspecific protection that doesn't differ based on threat; there is no recall or memory. But B-cells and T-cells involved in the adaptive immune response can learn to respond to new threats and recall those responses as needed. B-cells and T-cells are two different types of specialized white blood cells. The "B" originates from studying these cells in the bursa sac of chickens. The "T" comes from the origin of these cells in the thymus.

Two basic cell types organize this response—T-cells and B-cells. T-cells are judges; they decide whether to respond to this evidence or ignore it, and they base judgments on the volume and quality of the evidence and on the memory of similar or previous cases. Just as there are different judges in a court system, there are different classes of T-cells.

Immature or naive T-cells (TH0) can mature along several different paths. Recently, researchers have shown that these paths are flexible or plastic, depending on the volume and duration of exposure to the foreign protein, as well as on environmental influences (vitamin D, vitamin A, epigenetic factors such as diet, and cytokines or cell messengers). The basic categories are TH1 (autoimmune reaction), TH2 (allergic reaction), TH17 (autoimmune reaction), and Treg (regulatory T-cells, tolerance).

B-cells are the enforcers. Sometimes they present evidence, and other times they simply respond when other cells tell them what to target and round up. The T-cells can activate the B-cells into making specific antibodies that fight these pieces of evidence, or they themselves can transform and kill the invaders (abnormal cells). Vitamin D regulates the production of antibodies in this response.

Activated vitamin D suppresses and prevents the differentiation of native T-cells (TH0) into TH1, TH2, or TH17 cells in preference for the regulatory T-cell phenotype (Treg). Suppression of D-cell activation by vitamin D in the thymus (T-cell gland) and the peripheral lymph tissue (especially, gut-associated lymph tissue) and the presence of TGFβ and IL-10 drive the T regulatory phenotype. This regulatory response is necessary to the development of tolerance and the prevention of autoimmunity.

Vitamin D plays a key role in suppressing dendritic cell activity and subsequent T-cell maturation to establish tolerance to the self and the environment. Vitamin D influences the numbers of iNKT cells available to remember and suppress any inflammatory response to the self and a friendly environment. Vitamin D is also crucial in first-line defense against microorganisms by ensuring mucous membrane integrity, early recognition of pathogens, and clearance of invading organisms or abnormal cells.

The Perfect Storm

Vitamin D deficiency may produce autoimmunity through several different mechanisms, including the following:

1. Failure of tolerance during fetal development
2. Failure to develop tolerance to foods and normal bacteria (microbiome) in early and late childhood
3. Failure to clear infection, leading to chronic or recurrent infection
4. Loss of peripheral tolerance to foods or microbiome in adulthood and as you age
5. Any combination of 1 through 4

The failure of tolerance means your immune system begins to attack you sometimes—and even attack itself. This attack causes the release of numerous inflammatory substances (cytokines), including interferon, IL-1, IL-6, IL-17, TNF, prostaglandins, and many others. This swirl of inflammation feeds back on itself to produce a cyclone that wreaks havoc on your tissues.

Add to this picture the major role that your diet and acid-base balance play in regulating the immune response. Calcium in the wrong place promotes inflammation. Vitamins D and K help direct calcium traffic in and out of cells appropriately. Magnesium, citrates, and bicarbonates from vegetables and fruit raise the pH and suppress levels of inflammation. Animals need normal magnesium levels to fight off infection successfully. In their absence, the forecast calls for a downpour of cytokines.

Saturated fats stimulate your immune system, creating more inflammatory substances that raise the level of background inflammation, making it hard for the immune system to separate the good from the bad. On the other hand, omega-3 fats reduce the production of inflammatory substances in animals and humans. Omega-3 fats produce tolerance by helping to eliminate autoimmune T-cells, and omega-3 fats work side by side with vitamin D in the nucleus, where they regulate gene expression.

Acid excess hinders the ability of vitamin D to suppress D-cell activation. This may help if you have an abscess or a wound, but if you're facing an autoimmune disease, it is likely that acid excess feeds the inflammatory process by letting D-cells activate at will. When your body is in a state of acidosis, D-cells show a tenfold greater ability to present evidence of all kinds, which means your D-cells are activating willy-nilly. This out-of-control process probably makes you more likely to develop autoimmune disease and have it grow worse.

Type 1 Diabetes

Type 1 diabetes—also called juvenile diabetes—stems from antibodies directed to the islet cells in the pancreas. The islet cells make insulin in response to rising glucose levels in the blood. The inflammation these antibodies create eventually destroys the islet cells, causing diabetes. This differs from the insulin resistance of type 2 diabetes.

In the Netherlands thirty years ago, public health officials recommended rickets prevention with 2,000 IU of vitamin D a day (via cod-liver oil) from birth through a child's first birthday. In 1997, Dr. Elina Hyppönen and her colleagues at the Tampere School of Public Health in Finland analyzed health records of babies who were born in 1966 in Oulu and Lapland, Finland, to check for development of type 1 diabetes. This landmark analysis showed an 80 percent reduction in occurrence of type 1 diabetes among those who were receiving vitamin D at 2,000 IU per day. Those in the study who didn't take vitamin D and developed rickets as children had a 200 percent higher risk than compliant children of developing type 1 diabetes.

Unfortunately, this evidence didn't make a big impression on the Finns. Over the past forty years, the amount of D supplementation recommended in Finland has decreased from 2,000 to 400 IU per day, and more cases of type 1 diabetes resulted.

Vitamin D can prevent the development of type 1 diabetes if fetuses and young children have adequate levels of D while the immune system is developing. It all starts during fetal development when D-cells introduce islet-cell proteins to T-cells and scream "protection needed!" But lacking sufficient vitamin D to suppress these D-cells or to dumb down this interaction, the T-cells spur B-cells to make antibodies to the islet cells. These antibodies trigger an inflammatory response, which activates more D-cells and M-cells in the pancreas and the lymph system. As more and more islet-cell proteins are presented to more and more T-cells, the process expands—and eventually, this heightened anti-islet-cell response destroys them, which results in declining insulin production and diabetes development.

The sooner you normalize your vitamin D levels, the sooner you can halt this destructive cycle. The earlier in life your body has vitamin D on its side, the more islet-cell function you preserve. The take-home message is that all pregnant women badly need normal vitamin D levels throughout pregnancy.

Systemic Lupus Erythematosis

Systemic lupus erythematosis—simply called lupus—is an autoimmune disease that occurs when D-cells are randomly activated and proceed to jump-start T-cells that, in turn, instruct B-cells to make antibodies to *you*. Your body turns on you.

If you have lupus, your body may make antibodies to a variety of self-proteins, including skin, joints, muscles, kidneys, blood cells, and brain. These antibodies cause inflammation that can lead to organ damage.

Lupus sufferers often develop rashes, fever, enlarged lymph nodes, blood abnormalities, headaches, joint pain, and joint swelling. Occasionally, they have persistent chest pain, blood clots, kidney or nervous system inflammation.

The most typical course of lupus is a start-up during female adolescence or childbearing years when female hormones are cycling. Lupus is rare in postmenopausal women and in men. Estrogen and prolactin probably play important roles in the development of lupus. Estrogen combined with interferon spurs D-cells to develop into activated inflammatory cells rather than staying naive and tolerant. Counteracting this, vitamin D has been shown to suppress the estrogen signal and may delay the onset of puberty.

But lupus probably has its earliest origins during fetal development and/or childhood, when many scavenger cells are primed with self-evidence. At puberty, the rise in estrogen levels, combined with continued vitamin D deficiency, leads to rapid expansion of these scavenger populations primed to activate T-cells against self-evidence. Activated mature scavengers produce lots of interferon, which excites both T-cells and B-cells. It's only a matter of time before enough T-cells and B-cells are activated that disease shows up; in effect, your immune system has turned against you.

Doctors and researchers regularly see significantly lower vitamin D levels in people with lupus compared to those without this disease. We also know that lupus occurs more often in people with a great deal of melanin in their skin—and, as we've seen, these same people have trouble sustaining healthy vitamin D levels because of the sunscreen effect of that extra load of melanin.

In the United States, the number of cases of lupus is about 81 per 100,000 in European Americans, 375 per 100,000 in African Americans. Similarly, the prevalence in Afro Caribbeans who live in England is 251 per 100,000. This compares to 117 per 100,000 population in Afro Caribbeans in Curaçao in the West Indies, relatively near the equator.

Afro Caribbeans who move away from equatorial sunshine increase their risk of lupus by 200 percent.

Interferon—an inflammatory substance that a variety of white cells release, often in response to infections—drives the proliferation of the scavengers that present evidence of self- and foreign proteins in lupus. These activated scavenger cells then begin to produce their own interferon, which activates more scavengers. In essence, they activate themselves. In the absence of vitamin D, there is little to suppress this amplifying feedback loop. Administering activated vitamin D suppresses the production of interferon from these activated scavengers (D-cells). But the critical time for intervention/prevention is during pregnancy and in early childhood.

Multiple Sclerosis

In multiple sclerosis (MS), the immune system makes antibodies to proteins found in the nerve covering (the myelin sheath). The inflammation that results disrupts the nerve covering, which needs to be intact to speed transmission of electrical impulses. Disrupting the covering greatly slows transmission of electrical impulses, resulting in partial or permanent loss of sensation or muscle function.

In studying worldwide populations, Dr. John Kurtzke of the Veterans Administration Hospital in Washington, D.C., saw more cases of MS in places far removed from the equator, except for those places where people eat a great deal of cold-water fish, which is rich in vitamin D and omega-3 fats—Icelanders, for example.

If you were born and lived (prior to adolescence) above 37 degrees north latitude, your risk of MS is two to four times higher than if you had spent your childhood below 37 degrees north latitude. Furthermore, if you migrate from an equatorial climate with low risk to America or England, where MS is more common, the risk for the next generation will rise to the level of where you've relocated.

It's likely that your risk of developing MS is determined during fetal development and childhood, while your immune system is developing in the presence of vitamin D deficiency. Theories based on migration data suggest that an infectious agent may play a role in causing MS, but it's probably a combination of these factors. Remember that vitamin D deficiency increases your risk of infection at all ages.

The Nurses Health Study (Harvard University, 2004) showed a 40 percent reduction in the risk of MS among nurses whose intake of supplemental vitamin D was at least 400 IU per day. These results were confirmed in a 2006 study of U.S. military personal, when Harvard University researchers found that D levels at or above 40 in subjects younger than twenty years had the greatest impact on risk reduction. This confirms the importance of early exposure to adequate vitamin D to prevent autoimmune disease.

Additionally, studies on vitamin D supplementation in people with MS showed reduced disease activity when they began taking vitamin D supplements.

Inflammatory Bowel Disease

IBD can result from

- overgrowth of inflammatory bacteria that cause inflammation in the wall of the intestines (*E. coli, Salmonella, Shigella*);
- lack of tolerance to the normal healthy bacteria in the intestine;
- exposure to substances that inflame the bowel wall and destroy the intestinal barrier to bacteria (celiac disease).

The common denominator here is bacteria in the intestine. After you're born, microorganisms teach your immune system what's friendly and what's threatening with regard to viruses, bacteria, and fungi. The bugs in your gut also stimulate the production of a whole host of hormones that affect growth and development. "Bugs" means bacteria and some fungus (but *not* viruses).

Your relationship with the bacteria in your intestines influences everything from height and weight to heart, kidney, and lung capacity. How you interact with these bacteria and what bacteria actually grow determine whether you develop inflammatory bowel disease.

Healthy bacteria in the bowels are your partners—essentially, a *part* of you. When you develop inflammatory bowel disease, it's because your body failed to tolerate these healthy bacteria or other proteins in your intestines.

If you got IBD because of bacterial overgrowth, your bowel contents were contaminated by either invasive bacteria from food poisoning (*E. coli, S. typhi*) or unfriendly bacteria that grew wildly because of bad diet.

In a normal scenario, contaminated foods will give you fever, inflammation, bloody stools, and diarrhea, but after your body clears the invasive bacteria, those symptoms disappear.

Abnormalities in the immune system also can cause bowel inflammation. That's what happens with Crohn's disease and ulcerative colitis. A genetic predisposition teams up with failed tolerance, and you're left with chronic recurrent bowel inflammation. Your immune system can't handle the bacteria in your intestines, so the bowel lining becomes a battleground where the immune system is constantly attacking bacteria that attach to it. It's like you have an infected rash inside your gut.

Animals with vitamin D deficiency are more susceptible to gut damage from toxins and bacteria.

Supplementation of vitamin D in genetically altered mice prevents the development of IBD, and the treatment of diseased animals with additional activated vitamin D clears their inflammation and enhances gut repair.

Another way your immune system balks is by developing an inflammatory reaction in your bowels when exposed to certain proteins; this is much like an allergy. One of the most common proteins the intestine doesn't tolerate well is gluten, which is found in wheat, barley, rye, and sometimes oats. At least 1 percent of the world's population is gluten intolerant. If you are allergic and you continue to eat gluten, your small intestine stays inflamed.

The chronic D deficiency that results from poor absorption due to the inflammation in the small intestine may then predispose you to autoimmune diseases among the many other problems associated with D deficiency. Many people with celiac disease also have deficiencies of potassium, magnesium, iron, and vitamins A, K, and B. If you have recurrent canker sores or irritable bowel syndrome and other bowel symptoms, see a doctor for an evaluation.

Psoriasis

Psoriasis is a skin disease that causes patches of silvery, scaling skin that build up on a red base. Patches commonly occur on the scalp, elbows, knees, feet, and buttocks, but they can show up just about anywhere. Many people with psoriasis have abnormal nail growth, eye and joint inflammation, and intestinal inflammation.

Psoriasis typically starts before age twenty, but it can occur any time throughout life. Many different forms occur, but all appear to have the same cause. Current theories suggest that poor tolerance of bacteria (usually strep) on the skin, in the mouth, or in the nose triggers the immune response that leads to psoriasis.

For decades we've known that psoriasis gets worse in the winter and improves in the summer. This seasonal variation in disease activity has to do with UV light exposure and vitamin D production in the skin. In fact, doctors have traditionally treated psoriasis patients with ultraviolet light therapy and topical steroids.

In the past two decades, researchers have seen that activated vitamin D and vitamin D analogs applied as ointments can reduce or eliminate psoriasis—and enhance the effectiveness of ultraviolet light therapy. Activated vitamin D combined with a vitamin A compound is even more effective.

For centuries people have sunbathed in the Dead Sea as a remedy for skin diseases. The high magnesium content of Dead Sea water is the healing factor. This was proven by German scientists who studied cell activity in the skin of psoriasis patients and found that skin soaked with magnesium decreased the ability of scavenger cells to present proteins to the T-cells for activation. In other words, in the Dead Sea location, magnesium and UV light worked together to suppress immune cell activation in the skin of psoriasis patients.

Dr. Peter Mayser at Justus Liebig University in Giessen, Germany, treated psoriasis with intravenous omega-3 fatty acids and found that two types of psoriasis responded much better to those infusions than they did to omega-6 fat infusions.

A nutritious diet and vitamin D tend to "quiet" your immune system so it doesn't overreact to foreign proteins that come in contact with the skin.

Rheumatoid Arthritis

Rheumatoid arthritis is an autoimmune disease that causes arthritis in the small and large joints and also can cause inflammation in the eyes, lungs, and blood vessels. This disease worsens rapidly, leading to deformity and disability in only a few years unless the rheumatoid arthritis sufferer takes potent anti-inflammatory medications.

Doctors see rheumatoid arthritis in more women than men, three to one. Typically, sufferers are thirty to fifty, but you can have rheumatoid arthritis at any time from adolescence to age one hundred.

The Iowa Women's Health Study showed that women who took vitamin D supplements were less likely to develop rheumatoid arthritis. In three of five studies that used vitamin D or activated vitamin D to treat rheumatoid arthritis, researchers saw improvements in symptoms. People newly diagnosed with inflammatory arthritis had more severe disease the lower their vitamin D levels.

Animal studies examining inflammatory arthritis also show reduced inflammation in the joints when activated D was administered. Furthermore, when animals got activated vitamin D when they were immunized with collagen, it prevented joint inflammation.

Infections

Vitamin D and a good diet help your immune system develop clear memories of infectious agents and vaccines for effective defense. Recent studies from several universities demonstrate that vitamin D is required for adequate production of antimicrobial proteins from immune cells in response to infection. These proteins, as their name implies, kill bacteria. In the absence of these proteins, antibiotics are less effective, increasing the risk of resistance and chronic or recurrent infection.

UVB is essential for vitamin D synthesis, but it also can inactivate viruses. Low UVB levels in winter and falling vitamin D levels allow more viruses to hang around and make you more vulnerable to them. Flu is a perfect example: the peak of the flu season follows the summer solstice by six months, and its global spread alternates between the Northern and Southern hemispheres, in keeping with hemispheric seasonal changes.

Vitamin D levels reach their seasonal low in about March and into April and May as you move farther from the equator, which extends the flu season. Older people and children, who are most susceptible to severe influenza infection, often are the very people with vitamin D and dietary deficiencies.

A study published in *Pediatrics* in 2011 showed that low umbilical cord blood levels of vitamin D were associated with an increased risk of respiratory syncytial virus (RSV) related bronchiolitis through the first year of life. This means that low vitamin D levels during your mother's late pregnancy increase your risk of infection during the first year of your life.

Other major sources of serious infections in the United States—hospitals and nursing homes—are responsible for most complications, costs, and deaths due to hospitalization. We know that institutionalized people are at very high risk for vitamin D deficiency due to lack of sun exposure. Hospital-acquired infections are four times more common in African Americans and others with high melanin content.

Most people with HIV have low levels of both vitamin D and activated vitamin D. The role vitamin D plays in increasing a person's susceptibility to HIV infection is unclear, but the role that vitamin D plays in fighting tuberculosis (TB) and probably hepatitis C and other opportunistic viral and bacterial infections that AIDS patients suffer is indisputable.

Cranking Out Protection

Your immune system keeps churning away at its three big jobs throughout your life—functions that affect all the systems in your body. This amazing system protects you from infections, identifies and repairs damaged tissues, and forages for abnormal cells.

Most of the cells in your immune system have vitamin D receptors, so vitamin D affects their function. The receptors are just sitting there, waiting for feedback from D.

Vitamin D enhances the precision of D-cell judgment calls and ensures adequate NKT cell numbers. Vitamin D suppresses D-cell activation to ensure tolerance early in development. But later in childhood and when you're grown, it revs up your immune response with antimicrobial proteins to protect you from infections.

Autoimmune diseases such as type 1 diabetes, multiple sclerosis, and lupus are diseases in which tolerance has failed, and vitamin D deficiency appears to be the culprit behind this failure. Susceptibility to chronic or recurrent infections such as tuberculosis, hepatitis C, HIV, and even influenza and pneumonia all have ties to D-deficiency.

It's smart to simplify your life by giving your immune system a big boost via the Vitamin D Cure.

Lowering Your Risk

The recommendations in the Vitamin D Cure are estimated to lower your risk of autoimmune diseases by 50 to 90 percent depending on how early in childhood normalization of vitamin D and lifestyle changes occur. The earlier in pregnancy the changes occur, the lower the risk of autoimmunity for that new life. Recent information on the role of vitamin D in protecting us from infections suggests a 50 percent reduction in the risk of respiratory infections with fortification of vitamin D and diet.

12

The Vitamin D Cure
to Help Prevent
and Treat Cancer

Cancer means that your cell growth and differentiation have stopped responding to your body's usual control signals. Call them cells gone wild. But vitamin D does several things to keep this from happening. It

- slows the cell life cycle;
- stimulates tumor suppressor genes;
- partners with growth factors to promote normal differentiation;
- facilitates programmed cell death in abnormal cells;
- suppresses blood flow to tumors.

The development of cancer is something like the *I Love Lucy* assembly-line episode in which Lucy and Ethel tried to process chocolate candies that were coming down the conveyor belt so fast they couldn't be handled. One mistake was compounded by another. And that's essentially what happens to produce cancer cells. One mistake is followed by another until the cell production process flies totally out of control. If you could slow the speed of the assembly line, each member of your production team would have more time to complete his task and make fewer mistakes.

Cells are like assembly lines. Slow down the cell life cycle, and your body will have fewer errors in cell function and genetic replication, which will reduce the likelihood of malignant transformation. That's the point of no return, when enough critical errors occur that a cell becomes cancerous because it no longer responds to normal regulation.

We know that vitamin D slows a cell's life cycle, which is good because this means that the D lets fewer cells replicate their DNA and divide. Your cells make fewer errors because they have the time and the resources to correct their few errors.

The problem is, cells have a limited capacity to fix those errors in DNA replication. In part, vitamin D controls the genes and enzymes that can repair errors. Further, if errors slip past your body's quality-control officers, vitamin D may help to ensure that the bad parts or defective cells are destroyed, as a last-ditch form of quality control.

Dr. William Grant of the SUNARC Foundation in San Francisco, California, looked at the risk of cancer and death from cancer in relation to latitude and ultraviolet B (UVB) exposure in several global regions. In those who lived closer to the equator, Dr. Grant consistently found a lower risk for contracting and dying from a variety of cancers, including breast, prostate, colon, pancreatic, lymphoma, and lung cancer. The more sun, the lower the person's risk of dying of cancer. He also studied the risk of getting cancer as it relates to latitude/sun exposure and found a decreased risk of having many of the same cancers listed previously in people living close to the equator.

A recent blinded forward-looking study seems to confirm that vitamin D is the key ingredient here. Dr. Joan Lappe, of Creighton University in Nebraska, looked at the ability of vitamin D and calcium to prevent bone fractures in older women and found a 77 percent reduction in the appearance of any cancer from the first to the fourth year of follow-up among women taking 1,100 IU of vitamin D and 1,500 mg of calcium daily. This degree of benefit wasn't seen in the patients who were taking calcium only. (A blind forward study is the best investigative process because both patient and provider are blind to the treatment—active versus placebo. This study was prospective—treat and then follow patients—rather than retrospective: an analysis of an old database in search of patterns.)

The influence of diet on cancer risk is sometimes confusing. In general, you can lower your risk of gastrointestinal cancers if you eat fewer processed foods that are high in salt and saturated fat and low in fiber and if you increase your intake of fresh vegetables (particularly green, leafy vegetables) and fruits. But when you try to examine an isolated component of this diet, such as fiber or fat, no relationship is apparent.

The message is that you need to eat the actual foods because it's the exposure to "the whole package"—all the other elements in those foods over long periods of time—that produces health benefits. Supplements aren't a substitute for a healthy diet. They *help* but they don't replace good food.

Breast Cancer

Breast cancer—the second most common cancer in women behind nonmelanoma skin cancer—is the second leading cause of death among American women, behind lung cancer.

Your risk of breast cancer increases with age and obesity. And you're more likely to die of breast cancer if you're African American than if you're European American.

These findings are consistent with findings that cite a lower risk of breast cancer with increased ultraviolet light exposure, which means higher vitamin D levels are protective.

Before the first edition of *The Vitamin D Cure* was written, evidence from the Nurses Health Study suggested that lower estimated levels of vitamin D were associated with an increased risk of breast cancer, especially in postmenopausal women. This relationship wasn't confirmed, however, when researchers studied blood levels several years later.

Since then, a number of studies have shown a higher risk for developing breast cancer in postmenopausal women with low blood levels of vitamin D. Studies in women of various geographical locations seem to show a strong relationship between low vitamin D levels and more aggressive types of breast cancer with a poor prognosis, especially in premenopausal women.

With the discovery of breast cancer–associated gene mutations (BRCA1 and BRCA2), which dramatically increase the risk for getting breast cancer, many women thought a cure might be just around the corner. However, researchers detect these mutations in only about one in three hundred to five hundred people—and they account for less than 10 percent of breast cancers. To lesser degrees, these gene mutations also increase the risks of cancer of the ovaries, prostate, pancreas, and stomach and the risks of melanoma.

These genes play a fundamental role in cancer suppression. There are numerous tumor-suppressing genes, and when they mutate or something impairs their expression, cancer risk goes up. Tumor-suppressing genes actually have overlapping functions that reduce the risk of cancer development, and local/on-demand production of activated vitamin D turns on many of these genes, including BRCA1.

Activated vitamin D produced in breast tissue, including breast cancer cells, not only stimulates the production of tumor-suppressor genes, but it also directly increases the production of these proteins to slow the cell cycle at critical checkpoints. Pausing at these checkpoints allows other systems to repair problems or mutations before proceeding to the next phase of the cell cycle.

This pausing also slows the proliferation of breast cancer cells. In normal breast cells, this pause spurred by activated vitamin D (in conjunction with other growth factors) promotes normal differentiation of breast tissue.

If mutations aren't corrected or if a cell has already undergone malignant transformation, activated vitamin D can team up with other proteins to stimulate programmed death of abnormal cells.

Recent research shows that vitamin D suppresses the production of estrogen and its receptors in breast cancer cells. This is probably another way in which vitamin D slows breast cancer cell growth.

This evidence, along with animal studies, suggests that a girl who lacks adequate vitamin D during puberty years will have abnormal breast development. This, in turn, may increase a woman's susceptibility to risk factors such as alcohol for breast cancer development. In other words, the window of greatest opportunity for vitamin D to reduce breast cancer risk may be during childhood and puberty.

Prostate Cancer

Prostate cancer—the most common cancer besides skin cancer—is the number two cause of cancer death in men (lung cancer is number one). Here's what we know about prostate cancer risks:

- Your risk increases with age.
- African American men are 65 percent more susceptible to prostate cancer than European American men.
- Americans are twice as likely to die from it.
- A nonsmoking man has a higher risk of having prostate cancer than the risk of having cancers of the lung, colon, rectum, mouth, bladder, lymph system, and kidney combined.

Lower vitamin D levels increase your risk of developing and dying from prostate cancer. The risk of prostate cancer in European Americans increases in places farther from the equator, particularly north of the fortieth parallel. Studies on different measures of lifetime ultraviolet exposure show a lower risk of prostate cancer in people who get greater UV exposure. Since African Americans typically have vitamin D levels that are much lower than those of European Americans, this explains in part why African Americans have a much higher risk of death from prostate cancer.

When Japanese immigrated to the United States after World War II, the first and second generations of Japanese in the United States experienced quadruple the rate of prostate cancer compared to their native

Japanese counterparts. More recently, researchers have cited Westernization of diets and decreased intake of cold-water fish high in omega-3 fats and vitamin D as partial reasons for rising rates of prostate cancer in Japanese and Koreans.

Vitamin D suppresses tumor growth and promotes differentiation in prostate cancer similar to the way it works with breast cancer. In prostate cancer cell lines, vitamin D stimulates the tumor-suppressor genes that increase the production of proteins that slow the cell life cycle.

Vitamin D in prostate cancer cell lines increases the concentration of growth factors that promote normal division of prostate cells. Conversely, vitamin D decreases the concentrations of growth factors that speed cell life cycles.

Doctors find vitamin D receptors in higher concentrations in normal prostates than in enlarged prostates or in prostate cancer. In other words, normal prostate tissue is more likely to respond to vitamin D signals for normal growth and development. Benign enlarged prostates have about half as many vitamin D receptors as normal prostates, and prostate cancer cells have a tenth as many vitamin D receptors.

Apparently, abnormal prostates have less capacity to produce "on demand" activated vitamin D. Interestingly, in rodents, the concentration of vitamin D and testosterone receptors in different parts of the prostate is heavily influenced by the testosterone–vitamin D balance during preadolescent development. Again, the influence of vitamin D on early development may have a profound influence on disease development in adults, especially when you add dietary deficiencies to the mix.

Unlike breast tissue, the prostate gland is often inflamed in the years preceding enlargement and the development of cancer. Researchers at Stanford University hypothesize that this inflammation contributes to the gradual development and progression of cancer in the prostate and that vitamin D may be the perfect tool to decrease this inflammation. Prostate cancer cells produce prostaglandins. In this scenario, vitamin D suppresses prostaglandin production.

Vitamin D also shuts off two important nuclear factors (p38 MAPK and NF-KB) that promote the production of numerous inflammatory and angiogenic (blood flow–increasing) substances (see chapter 11). A small study at Stanford University testing this theory in prostate cancer patients who used active vitamin D and naproxen showed a slowing of the growth of prostate cancer in three-quarters of the patients.

Clinical research on activated vitamin D and vitamin D–like molecules in humans shows promise. We know that activated vitamin D alone often slows the growth of prostate tumors, and the different concentrations of vitamin D receptors on cancer cells versus normal prostate cells can help to separate cancer cells from normal cells by growth rates. This separation allows doctors to use conventional chemotherapy more effectively to kill cancer cells.

Colorectal Cancer

Colon cancer—the third-leading cause of cancer in men and women combined when skin cancer is excluded—is today's third-biggest cause of death related to cancer.

Thanks to increased education on colon cancer and a growing number of colonoscopy screenings, the number of deaths from colon cancer has dropped in the past fifteen years. But this cancer remains a big problem, and one that people want to know more about so they can prevent its occurrence if possible.

To work toward prevention, you need to understand the process of colon cancer development. You have large amounts of bacteria in your colon and rectum but very little in the mouth and stomach. If your stomach is functioning normally and producing acid that's not blocked by medications, much of the bacteria in your food is killed before it can enter the small intestine.

Limiting the growth of bacteria in the small intestine are gallbladder bile acids, pancreatic enzymes, and rapid transit. The movement of food from your mouth to your anus takes two to three days, but only four to six hours of this time are spent between the mouth and the entrance to the colon. This means that your digested food spends about two days in the colon and rectum, and that's where all the bacteria selected in the first part of digestion can begin to grow.

Your immune system has a delicate relationship with these bacteria that starts at birth, when bacteria are introduced to your intestine. For one thing, we know that breast-fed infants have a different profile of bugs in their intestine that are friendlier and less often associated with infections and disease than the profile of bugs in formula-fed infants. This is important because if the relationship between your immune system and the bugs doesn't go well, that glitch can lead to diseases such as inflammatory bowel disease, polyps, and colon cancer.

Vitamin D in the immune system stimulates the production of proteins that kill viruses and bacteria, and specialized cells in the intestines also can make these substances, which are partly vitamin D–regulated. If unfriendly strains of bacteria begin to grow in the intestine, they will trigger an immune response that clears them and vitamin D is part of this response.

But if you're deficient in vitamin D, this killing/clearing process is flawed, as in the case of tuberculosis. You're hit with unfriendly strains of bacteria, and your body lets them hang around to give you trouble. On the other hand, if you got the bacteria from food, continuing to consume the foods or medicines that pave the way for bad bugs will serve to keep them around.

The presence of unfriendly bacteria produces ongoing inflammation, which speeds the colonic cell life cycle, increasing the chances of DNA errors and malignant transformation. This means you're more likely to end up with cancer.

People with inflammatory bowel disease, especially ulcerative colitis, have a high risk of developing colon cancer because of the chronic inflammation in the intestine. Similarly, people who are chronically infected with the ulcer-causing bacteria *H. pylori* are at increased risk for certain types of stomach cancer.

Nonsteroidal anti-inflammatory drugs in high doses reduce the development of polyps in the intestines by reducing inflammation.

Vitamin D plays an important role in regulating and defining your immune system's response to bacteria in the intestine, as well as in enhancing the integrity of mucous membranes in the gut. Your diet can either foster the growth of friendly bacteria or feed the proliferation of unfriendly bacteria that will lead to inflammation and perhaps produce cancer-causing substances. Diet and vitamin D seem to influence your risk of bowel cancer more than your risk of other cancers.

In 1980, Drs. Frank and Cedric Garland of the University of California at San Diego reported his observations that a lack of UV exposure may make a person more likely to develop colon cancer. This was based on an analysis of death rates from colon cancer that showed the highest mortality in states with the lowest solar radiation. Since then, we've seen similar results in many studies analyzing UV exposure, vitamin D levels, and rates of colon and rectal cancer, or death from colon cancer.

Vitamin D suppresses tumor growth and promotes normal differentiation in colorectal cancer cells in much the same ways it does in breast and prostate cancer. Normal colon cells have higher vitamin D receptor concentrations than abnormal or cancerous colon cells.

Skin Cancer

Skin cancer is the most common form of cancer in both men and women. Usually people lump all skin cancers together, but significant differences exist in frequency and prognosis for different skin cancers.

The most common skin cancer is basal cell, which accounts for about 80 percent of skin cancers; next most common are squamous cell cancers. Melanomas are the least common. Of more than 2 million new cases of skin cancer a year, only 68,130 are melanoma. Of those 68,130, only 16 percent are invasive. Seventy-four percent of skin-cancer deaths are attributed to malignant melanoma.

UV light is one of about sixty carcinogens that the World Health Organization recognizes. Evidence that links UV exposure to basal cell and squamous cell cancer of the skin is plentiful and indisputable.

But melanoma has a more chameleon image. Recent studies on UV index, latitude, and incidence of melanoma have shown an increase in the risk of melanoma with increasing UV index and decreasing latitude, but only in white, non-Hispanic populations. In populations of color, researchers see no clear relationship to sun exposure. In fact, African Americans are usually diagnosed at a later stage and have a worse prognosis than European Americans. Even so, ultraviolet light does seem to be involved in the cause of most skin cancers.

Three decades ago, researchers told us that indoor workers were at greater risk of melanoma skin cancer than outdoor workers and that people who worked in jobs that had indoor and outdoor components were at the lowest risk of melanoma.

This made some experts wonder about the sun link to melanoma, especially since we've long known that some of the most common melanoma skin lesion sites are non-sun-exposed areas of the body. This suggests that some sun exposure may actually reduce the risk of melanoma.

The results of a National Cancer Institute study in 2004 indicate that you'll reduce your risk of developing melanoma if you take in larger amounts of vitamin D and vitamin A. In 2005, Dr. Marianne Berwick and colleagues at the University of New Mexico showed that patients with early-stage melanoma who had had more sun exposure had a lower risk of dying from melanoma. This told us that vitamin D may play a role in improved prognosis for melanoma patients. Furthermore, lab and animal studies on vitamin D and melanoma show that melanoma cells have D receptors and that activated vitamin D slows the growth of cells in culture and tumors in animals.

Perhaps the answer to preventing melanoma is *not* elimination of sun exposure through avoidance or the use of sunscreen. And that makes sense when you remember that we've been evolving under the sun for more than 2 million years. Maybe the sun isn't such a bad guy after all. The question remains—how much sun is enough? Is regular, intermittent exposure safer than long periods of no exposure followed by high exposure? What about the balance of UVA and UVB light?

Tanning certainly increases vitamin D levels, but how safe is tanning? We've seen that increasing solar UV exposure decreases the risk of more than a dozen different forms of cancer.

The news is that you can dance around this controversy altogether by just following the Vitamin D Cure. Supplementation is a perfect answer. It's safe to take vitamin D supplements based on your weight because you can simply monitor your blood levels—and with supplements, you certainly won't increase your risk of melanoma. Follow the advice in our sun-exposure charts in chapter 5 and you'll get adequate vitamin D without overexposure.

Diet and Cancer

How does your diet affect your likelihood of getting cancer? We know for sure that your entire diet is important—and that if you eliminate the "toxic" parts and ramp up the good parts, you'll reduce your risk of cancer. Large population studies repeatedly show that diets high in processed meat, salt, and saturated fat and low in vegetables, fruits, and fiber increase the risk of developing cancer, especially bowel cancer.

But when you separate individual components such as fiber or fat, you see no cancer/food relationship. For example, in 2000 the *New England Journal of Medicine* reported a study that found no effect from increasing cereal fiber on the recurrence of colorectal adenomas. Similar studies on fat intake and breast cancer in the Women's Health Initiative Study didn't show a relationship, either.

The problem is that all these variables taken together create other variables, adding up to a complex matrix of influencing factors. In the case of colon cancer, some of these additional variables are the bacteria that feed off your diet. If you change the recipe, you change the bacteria. But how many of the ingredients have to change before the bugs change? Are some ingredients more important than others? Do different combinations of ingredients favor completely different bacteria? With more than five hundred different species of bugs in your gut, the possibilities approach infinity.

The bacteria in your intestine provide additional nutrients from metabolism of food. They protect you from harmful bacteria by suppressing their growth. And they stimulate the growth and development of your organ systems, the most important of which is your immune system.

It's not easy to study the effects of diet on intestinal bacteria and then translate this into effects on specific diseases. We need more research to gain a fuller understanding of this relationship. Until then, it's clear that when you change your diet, you change the bacteria in your body, and that alters your risk for disease. The Vitamin D Cure is your easy recipe for healthy bacteria and for a healthy physical relationship with bacteria.

The Vitamin D Cure eating plan can be a helpful partner in your quest for health, or it can be a barrier. Give yourself a green light to lots of vegetables—the more, the better. They have the highest concentrations of antioxidants, vitamins, and minerals of any foods available today, minus the substances associated with cancer development, and they generate body-friendly bacteria. As a bonus, these foods contain almost no calories.

You can truthfully look at the Vitamin D Cure as the ultimate cancer-fighting agent. If you have cancer in your genetic code—as most of us do—take the reins and eat in a way that staves off cancer development.

The welcome facts are in. The right food is everywhere. All it takes is your own tweaking of your everyday diet. You don't have to overhaul everything you eat. Shoot for a 90 percent rate of doing the right stuff and you'll make a world of difference in your health and your body's propensity to develop cancer.

Lowering Your Risk

The recommendations in the Vitamin D Cure are estimated to lower your risk of most cancers by 50 percent. The science to support this is strongest for breast, colon, and prostate cancer. New information suggests that vitamin D may also lower your risk of skin cancer. Dietary changes are most effective at lowering the risk of bowel cancer.

13

The Vitamin D Cure
for Your Bones,
Joints, and Teeth

At first glance, the role of vitamin D in bone development seems obvious. Vitamin D builds bone. Or does it?

Vitamin D influences skeletal growth during the nine-month fetal period and your childhood years. The D hormone is important in all aspects of bone production. However, when you're calcium deficient due to an acidic diet or a lack of vitamin D, your activated vitamin D works to disintegrate or break down your bone to mobilize minerals and raise blood levels of calcium.

The role that vitamin D plays depends on where you are in your life cycle, your nutrition, and your health. During fetal development and childhood, vitamin D works in conjunction with growth hormone and sex steroids to build structurally sound bone. During adulthood, vitamin D regulates a balancing act between bone formation and bone breakdown. Vitamin D during child development is a bone-former, but in adults, it's a bone-turnover regulator.

Here are some vitamin D facts:

- You need vitamin D to heighten your muscle mass, strength, and coordination.

- You need vitamin D so your teeth will develop normally and stay healthy.

- Having sufficient vitamin D will reduce your calcium needs.

The Calcium Balancing Act

Calcium is important for strong bones. You've heard that anthem since you were a kid.

But that's not the whole story; it's actually the *balance* of calcium that is really important, not just how much you take. If you aren't absorbing it, or if you're losing it faster than you're taking it in, you still don't have enough.

The quality of your diet is the loose cannon that makes the difference in how calcium, vitamin D, and food work together to keep you healthy. What you eat regularly definitely affects the way vitamin D functions in your bones. Here's why:

1. Eating enough protein helps to maintain your bone and muscle mass.

2. Magnesium and omega-3 fats slow bone turnover.

3. Salt, cheese, and refined grains work against vitamin D function because they generate acidosis and inflammation that sap calcium, magnesium, and protein from your bones and muscles.

4. Green, leafy vegetables and other kinds of produce are big members of the vitamin D booster club; they balance acid-base and preserve bone and muscle mass.

Pain

Because I'm a rheumatologist, people come to see me because they want solutions for the pain they're experiencing in their joints, tendons, ligaments, muscles, and bones. They typically have at least one disease involving muscles, ligaments, joints, or bones, but all of the aches and pains they have are actually connected to their vitamin D levels and what they eat.

Brenda, for example, was sixty-three when she came to see me about the pain in her hands, especially at the ends of her fingers and the bases of her thumbs. Because her knuckles had enlarged in the years following menopause, she was worried that she was developing arthritis. Her mother's arthritis had led to horribly deformed fingers that made it impossible to engage in everyday activities. Brenda's knees were swollen and painful, with small amounts of fluid in them. Her CLINHAQII was 0–35–70–45–7 (function, pain, fatigue, health perception, sleep), with thirty minutes of morning stiffness, and her vitamin D level tested at 34 at the end of summer (her peak).

Brenda began the Vitamin D Cure, and when she returned to see me in three months, she felt so much better that she swore she would never return to her old ways of eating, even though the diet part of the Vitamin D Cure was hard for her. This time around, she posted much better CLINHAQII scores (0–20–40–20–7), no morning stiffness, and a vitamin D level of 60. Her symptoms had improved by 40 percent, and she accomplished this without medications and with no side effects and more benefits. The changes she made may slow progression of her arthritis.

Today in the United States, the leading causes of disabilities are muscle, bone, and joint diseases. Lower-back pain is number one.

We know that arthritis causes these symptoms more often in people with extra-high skin melanin—those who are more likely to be deficient in vitamin D because their skin melanin serves as sunscreen, preventing them from soaking up vitamin D as easily as people with less melanin. The 2002 National Health Interview Survey showed that

African Americans and Hispanics with arthritis have more problems with limited mobility, work limitations, and severe joint pain than European Americans with arthritis. Clearly, people with more skin melanin and a higher risk for vitamin D deficiency simply have more trouble with arthritis.

As the North American population ages and as people live longer, a greater number of us have osteoarthritis of the knees, back, and neck. Advanced age brings increased risk for vitamin D and nutritional deficiencies, but it's not true that as you age, you should simply expect to have arthritis.

SARAH'S SHOULDER AND HIP PAIN

Sarah, seventy, had been hurting for two years. Progressive pain in her shoulders and hips was accompanied by fatigue and sleep disturbance. She had gained ten pounds, and her fingernails had become brittle. She felt itchy but had no rash.

Her bones and muscles were very sensitive to touch, and her shins were extremely tender to pressure. She had the bony enlargement of finger joints that's common with osteoarthritis. Her general health was normal.

Sarah posted CLINHAQII scores of 0.125–55–85–50–8 (function, pain, fatigue, health perception, sleep); she felt stiff in the mornings for just a few minutes. Her lab tests showed normal general chemistries, blood counts, thyroid function, arthritis markers, and inflammatory markers. Her vitamin D level was 28, with normal PTH and calcium.

We started Sarah on vitamin D 27 IU per pound per day, a calcium supplement, and a magnesium supplement. We told her to avoid salt, cheese, and grains, and to eat fresh produce and lean protein in a 3:1 ratio.

Three months later, her CLINHAQII scores were 0–15–0–0–10, with no morning stiffness. Her vitamin D level was now 65. Her function had returned to normal. Her pain was more than 70 percent better. The fatigue was gone, and her sleep had improved. She no longer itched, and her nails looked more normal. Interestingly, when people take vitamin D supplementation, rashes and itching on lower extremities often resolve.

Sarah's experiences drive home the point that you can address vitamin D and dietary deficiencies at any age. Young children as well as senior adults respond dramatically to this program.

Osteoarthritis

Osteoarthritis affects about 10 percent of the U.S. population—about 30 million Americans. Osteoarthritis (OA)—classically described as degeneration of the cartilage in the knees—is what most people think of as simple "wear and tear." In other words, your cartilage is wearing out, so you're going to have pain, like it or not. There is some truth to this, but what's far more important is that certain precautions will keep you from developing osteoarthritis in the first place.

Genetics plays a role. If you're a woman and your mother had osteoarthritis in her hands, with bony nodules and deformity, you're more likely to have osteoarthritis than a woman who doesn't have this history of osteoarthritis—or a male. Also, if you have a family history of degenerative disc disease, your back pain is probably related to disc disease. At the same time, though, inherited or adopted lifestyle counts as well. Your genetics is only the first number in the combination that unlocks a disease; the remaining numbers are under your control.

To understand osteoarthritis, think of your body as a building that needs a foundation to support interlocking materials of framing, siding, and roofing. A foundation that moves or cracks disrupts the integrity of the building that sits on it. Similarly, the bone that lies under joint cartilage keeps the cartilage stable, functioning, and durable. It follows that you will speed up the rate of your cartilage breaking down when anything destabilizes the bone below the cartilage, such as poor bone development or increased bone turnover caused by vitamin D deficiency, menopause, inadequate omega-3 fatty acid intake, and/or dietary acid-base imbalance.

RITA'S MISERY REVERSED

Consider the story of Rita, seventy-six, who came to my office seeking help with enlarged joints and pain in her feet, hands, knees, and lower back. She had severe fatigue, headaches, and difficulty performing daily activities. By the afternoon of most days, her ankles and feet began to swell.

When I examined Rita, I saw enlarged knee bones, second toes, and finger joints. She could barely move her knees, and her ankles were swollen; clearly, she had osteoarthritis. Her CLINHAQII scores were 1.25–75–100–50–6 (function, pain, fatigue, health perception, sleep), and blood tests done in June (the start of summer) showed a vitamin D level of 22.

Rita started the Vitamin D Cure, and after a year of following the cure, she described dramatic resolution in her pain and fatigue. She no longer had swollen legs. Her CLINHAQII numbers were 0–40–0–0–6; her vitamin D level had climbed to 73. At the one-year follow-up, Rita told us she wouldn't need to come back again. She was well!

How Vitamin D Impacts Osteoarthritis

Scientists spent more than fifty years studying the health of residents of Framingham, Massachusetts, and when Dr. Timothy McAlindon of Tufts University analyzed some of the Framingham information, he saw a two- to threefold faster rate of osteoarthritis progression in people who were in the lowest 20 percent of vitamin D levels compared to those in the highest.

Since that initial observation, three large studies in three countries have confirmed that low vitamin D levels are associated with a much higher risk of osteoarthritis of the knees and the hips, especially in people with weak bones. This is consistent with laboratory and human studies showing increased markers of bone turnover below the cartilage in people with osteoarthritis.

The Framingham study tells us that the degree of osteoarthritis reflects the degree of overweight. As in heart disease and diabetes, obesity is a red flag for high insulin levels, low vitamin D levels, and high amounts of inflammation. These high levels of inflammation are the major driver of increased bone turnover that leads to osteoarthritis, and vitamin D plays an important role in suppressing that inflammation and turnover. If you are overweight, this all may sound like really bad news. You're having lots of leg or knee pain, and you need to lose weight to feel better. You also can look at it from the other side: this problem is fixable without too much trouble. Losing as little as 11 pounds reduces the symptoms of osteoarthritis of the knee by 50 percent.

A CDC National Health Interview Survey showed that 31 percent of obese Americans have arthritis, but only 15 percent of normal or underweight Americans have arthritis. These numbers are consistent with the Framingham study, which shows the risk of severe osteoarthritis doubling in those who are extremely obese.

Dr. Robin Christensen, at H. S. Fredriksberg Hospital in Denmark, compared the experiences of eighty people with osteoarthritis and obesity by giving forty of them a low-calorie diet and weekly counseling and the other half a control diet and a weight-loss pamphlet. The WOMAC (Western Ontario McMaster Arthritis Index) score, which measures symptoms and function in osteoarthritis patients, improved 9 percent for every 1 percent reduction in body weight, and a 28 percent improvement in function for every increment of 10 percent weight loss.

Optimizing D levels and increasing dietary potassium, magnesium, and omega-3 fatty acids may slow or stop progression of osteoarthritis by slowing bone turnover and cartilage disintegration. These interventions may even reverse some changes from disease. But if you get a jump on things and optimize these nutrients during fetal development and childhood, you probably can stave off these forms of arthritis altogether.

Gout and Pseudogout

If you have high levels of uric acid, you may suffer from the form of arthritis called gout. Compared to women, men produce more uric acid because of the lack of estrogen. But after women go through menopause and stop making estrogen, they start producing uric acid in amounts equal to those of men. That's why women seldom have gout before menopause, but later in life can have the same problems with it that men do.

Gout is one in a cluster of diseases called the "metabolic syndrome" (see chapter 9). Gout often accompanies obesity, high blood pressure, cholesterol abnormalities, and diabetes. Most people with the metabolic syndrome have high uric acid levels, but only some of these individuals go on to develop gout.

More than 9 million Americans have gout, and African Americans have twice the likelihood of developing gout as European Americans. The incidence of gout in Asians and Latin Americans is also slightly higher than in European Americans, probably because of the increased incidence of high blood pressure in these ethnic groups.

A diet that generates acid and raises insulin levels tends to raise uric acid levels. In addition, kidney function declines with chronic high blood pressure and age, leading to decreased elimination of uric acid in urine and higher uric acid levels in the blood. Overly high uric acid levels can crystallize in the joints and cause inflammation.

Gout causes intermittent pain and swelling in the toes, ankles, knees, elbows, fingers, and/or wrists. Gout also affects the spine, shoulders, and hips, but because these sites are more unusual for those with gout, the problem may go undiagnosed.

A similar disease, pseudogout ("false gout"), is another form of arthritis, but this one stems from calcium crystals in the cartilage and joint fluid. Vitamin D deficiency, metabolic acid-base imbalance, magnesium deficiency, and high PTH levels, among other metabolic problems, mobilize calcium from the bone beneath the cartilage in an effort to raise calcium levels. These calcium salts sometimes diffuse into the cartilage and the joint fluid, where they can cause inflammation.

A person can have both gout and pseudogout. Gout can affect men at any time after adolescence, but pseudogout typically hits after age fifty, in both men and women, when vitamin D levels often fall lower. Symptoms are pain, stiffness, and swelling in the knees, shoulders, wrists, fingers, feet, hips, and/or spine.

Because joint cartilage is like a sponge, it swells and becomes slimy and rubbery when it's wet with joint fluid. This lubricates your joints for movement. But cartilage also has a very limited blood supply and gets all of its nutrition from joint fluid, which is like serum or blood without the red blood cells. If your blood has a high uric acid level, it's high in joint fluid as well and in the cartilage that has soaked it up. Similarly, if low vitamin D and magnesium levels are making you lose calcium from the bone below the cartilage, the cartilage will soak up the released calcium and phosphate.

When uric acid and/or calcium salts crystallize, they do so in the cartilage as well as in the joint fluid, which makes the cartilage stiff and brittle. This cartilage won't function normally. Gout and pseudogout actually speed up the breakdown of cartilage in osteoarthritis.

The inflammation from these crystals causes swelling and pain—often called "inflammatory osteoarthritis." Flare-ups may be inflammation due to gout or pseudogout that hasn't been diagnosed yet. Often doctors fail to connect pseudogout to imbalanced vitamin D and diet. Making matters worse, inflammation from flare-ups accelerates bone turnover around the inflamed joint and magnifies the problem.

When surgeons operate on people with ruptured discs and osteoarthritis of the spine, they often find uric acid crystals and calcium crystals in the intervertebral disc and in material removed from the spine. This is especially true in arthritis involving the neck (these patients may have severe headaches and/or fever).

MARK'S STORY

Mark, forty-nine, came to see me seeking better control of gout symptoms. For the previous two years, he'd had intermittent swelling and pain in his toes and ankles that was becoming more frequent and intense. These episodes usually would last five days; ibuprofen helped the pain. Recently the attacks had been lasting longer and were more severe, leading to absences from work.

He weighed 200 pounds, with a BMI of 30, and his blood pressure was 155/102. His lab work revealed a uric acid level of 10.0 (the normal range is 3.9 to 8.3) and a vitamin D level of 37 in late May. We had Mark start the Vitamin D Cure and the medications colchicine and probenicid. These meds can help prevent acute gout attacks but usually don't lower uric acid by more than a point or so.

On his two-month follow-up visit, Mark had lost weight and improved his blood pressure. He now weighed 188 pounds, with a BMI of 28, and his blood pressure was 140/93. His uric acid was 6.5; his vitamin D level was 78. We attributed most of the uric acid improvement to dietary changes because he'd also had dramatic weight loss and decreased his blood pressure, neither of which should have been affected by the medications. At five months he had lost six more pounds, and his blood pressure was stable at 142/92. Mark hadn't experienced any gout attacks since his initial visit. The final plan: he was going to continue his new and improved diet and the vitamin D supplements; and he would see his family physician for further treatment of his elevated blood pressure.

Eating the right foods can help prevent gout and pseudogout. What affects the ability of uric acid and calcium salts to stay dissolved in liquid are:

- Your acid-base balance
- Your joint-fluid concentration of uric acid and calcium that's related to your state of hydration
- The presence of protein and the presence of other minerals in the joint fluid

Acid-base imbalance allows calcium crystals from the bone and cartilage to migrate into the joint fluid. Dehydration can increase the concentration of uric acid and calcium in the joint. In the joint fluid, these crystals lead to inflammation.

When Dr. Hyon Choi of Harvard analyzed diets of forty-seven thousand participants in the twelve-year Health Professions Study, he found that those in the top twentieth percentile of animal-meat intake (and particularly seafood intake) had 40 to 50 percent more gout attacks. In contrast, gout attacks dropped about 45 percent in those people who were in the top twentieth percentile of low-fat dairy intake (drinking two or more glasses of skim milk per day).

This same study showed that fruit-based beverages, including wine and fruit juices, either reduced or had no adverse effect on the frequency of gout attacks. In contrast, beverages derived from grain with little or no potassium or magnesium, such as beer and whiskey, increased the frequency of gout attacks significantly.

Additional findings from Dr. Choi and others show a direct relationship between the risk of gout and the number of high-fructose-corn-syrup-containing beverages consumed per day. In contrast, the more water you consume in twenty-four hours, the lower your risk of a gout attack.

Comparing the diets of people with gout to those without gout, researchers have seen that increased intake of fiber, folic acid, and vitamin C from vegetables and fruit leads to a significant reduction in the risk of gout. Surprisingly, the gout-free people who consumed more vegetables and fruits also consumed more meat and seafood than those with gout. So the right balance of produce and protein is critical to reducing uric acid levels and gout risk.

Metabolic acid-base imbalance from out-of-sync diets (insufficient protein and fresh produce and too much salt and grain) lowers your blood levels of potassium and magnesium. Lower magnesium levels spur pseudogout attacks. By the same token, you can resolve episodic arthritis attacks via vitamin D supplementation and an improved diet that replaces missing magnesium.

Simply put, gout and pseudogout attacks happen more often when your ratio of protein to fresh produce is off-kilter. When you eat an average amount of protein but fail to balance this with generous amounts of fresh produce—especially magnesium-containing green vegetables—the resulting acid-base imbalance creates conditions that are ripe for gout and pseudogout attacks. If you have vitamin D deficiency, that makes things worse by accelerating your bone and cell turnover, increasing the release of both calcium and uric acid from the bone, which makes it available for crystallizing in the joints.

Strength and Coordination Issues

Vitamin D, magnesium, and calcium play critical roles in normal muscle function. In severe vitamin D deficiency, you lack the ability to get calcium into your muscles for contraction and get calcium out quickly for relaxation of muscles. This leads to decreased power from poor contraction and impaired relaxation, which often produces symptoms such as cramping or twitching.

With severe vitamin D deficiency and metabolic acidosis, you become catabolic, breaking down bone and robbing muscle to mobilize alkaline minerals calcium and magnesium to restore acid-base balance. The upshot is weak muscles and reduced coordination. Higher vitamin D levels and supplementation are linked to increased power, improved relaxation, and enhanced coordination.

Dr. Heike Bischoff-Ferrari, at the University of Basel in Switzerland, led a group that gave either placebos or vitamin D 800 IU with calcium of 1,200 milligrams to 122 older women with an average age of eighty-five. During the twelve-week treatment, researchers saw a 49 percent reduction in the number of falls compared to what had occurred in the six weeks prior to treatment. Those who received vitamin D and calcium also showed greater strength compared to the group on placebos.

Many people lose the ability to sit, stand, or walk and begin to experience frequent falls because they've grown weaker and weaker. Tests have revealed severely depressed vitamin D levels and markedly elevated PTH levels in these people, and many of them had low blood calcium levels or severe calcium deficiency. But when the same folks took regimens of vitamin D and calcium supplements, they regained muscle strength and coordination in weeks and were able to sit, stand, and walk again.

Protein and Strength

It takes protein to make protein (muscle). If you don't eat enough protein to keep the brain, heart, and kidneys going, you end up robbing Peter to pay Paul. This sounds obvious, but it's often overlooked.

When an older person moves slowly using a cane, people presume that's from age-related weakness. But for elderly women in particular, malnutrition is a more likely explanation.

Dietary surveys consistently show that Americans sixty-five and older typically don't get enough protein or fresh produce. But this problem isn't limited to seniors. Young vegetarians sometimes seek medical help for pain, fatigue, and generalized weakness—some even have liver dysfunction—and their problem may well be inadequate protein.

Why Do Bones Break?

If you break a bone without a high-impact force involved (in a car accident or a fall from a cliff, for example), you can't assume that a trauma caused the break. Children fall many times a day and usually don't break bones; and adult bones are stronger so they shouldn't break under everyday stress.

The problem in adults is osteoporosis, a disease of the skeleton that involves changes in bone structure down to the microscopic level. The changes accumulate, and soon you have a higher risk of having bone failure and/or breakage.

The situation is set up early in life. The less protein, calcium, magnesium, and phosphorus incorporated into bone from fetal development through childhood, the higher your risk for osteoporosis and fractures later in life. The more rapidly your bone breaks down and gets replaced by new bone (bone turnover), the higher the risk for fracture.

Osteoporosis affects more than ten million Americans, eight million of whom are women older than fifty-five. However, more than 34 million Americans have low bone mass and are at risk for developing osteoporosis. African Americans have a slower rate of bone turnover due to genetics, and they also maintain a higher peak bone mass (the point of highest accumulation of bone in a lifetime), which lowers their risk of osteoporosis compared to European Americans.

You don't reach peak bone mass until several years after puberty is complete. But your peak may be predetermined long before that; construction of your skeleton in your mother's womb and early in child-hood probably presets your peak bone mass. Studies on vitamin D levels during pregnancy show decreased bone mass in children at nine years whose mothers were D-deficient while their babies were in the uterus.

A person who fails to meet her potential peak bone mass will have an increased fracture risk for a lifetime. Conversely, if you maximize the factors that enhance bone formation in childhood, it's likely you can prevent osteoporosis in adulthood.

Your children will reach their potential peak bone mass if you do the following:

- Maintain normal vitamin D levels during pregnancy.

- Make sure your children get enough vitamin D from diet, sun, and/or supplements.

- Provide your children with an acid-base-balanced diet that has adequate protein and omega-3 fatty acids.

- Make sure your kids do weight-bearing exercise starting as soon as they can walk. Playing sports outdoors, climbing trees, and riding bikes are all good activities for healthy bones.

To measure your bone density, you can have an X-ray test that uses less radiation than dental X-rays. It determines the amount of mineral in your bones—your bone mineral density, also called BMD or bone mass. Your test result is called a T-score—a measure of how far above or below you are compared to your peak bone mass.

What's interesting about this test is that the relationship between a bone mineral density test result and the risk of fracture is very close—closer, in fact, than the relationship between cholesterol and the risk of heart attack or between high blood pressure and the risk of stroke.

The U.S. government gives us averages that doctors can use as standards for calculating T-scores. Here's how the results break down:

- Negative T-score: your bones have less mineral than desirable, and your fracture risk is increased

- 0 to –0.9: normal

- –1.0 to –2.4: osteopenia or moderately low

- –2.5 or less: osteoporosis

- Higher than 0.0: your bones have more mineral than average

Don't be lulled into complacency and think you don't need to make any lifestyle changes because your BMD was "normal." A drop in bone density is a late finding in this whole process. Most of my patients with severe vitamin D and dietary deficiencies have normal BMDs, but they definitely don't have healthy bones. So don't wait to find out what your bone density is before taking action to build bone.

The lower your vitamin D levels, the lower your bone mass and the higher your potential fracture rate. Norway's Tromsø Study showed relationships among age, high PTH, low BMD, and high blood pressure in women. The older you are and the higher your PTH, the more likely you are to have low BMD and high blood pressure.

The Women's Health Initiative Study showed increased bone mass in hips when women had been taking as little as 400 IU of vitamin D plus calcium. Also, people with lower starting vitamin D levels seemed to respond better to supplementation.

A review of research looking at vitamin D treatment for osteoporosis published in the *Journal of the American Medical Association* showed an average 26 percent reduction in hip fractures and a 23 percent reduction in all nonspine fractures. This magnitude of protection exceeds the benefits seen with some medications currently approved by the FDA for the prevention and treatment of osteoporosis.

These benefits were seen only in studies using 800 IU per day or more of vitamin D. Studies that looked at lower doses showed no decrease in fracture rates. This emphasizes the need to normalize vitamin D levels rather than providing some universal dosing for vitamin D.

Protein for Good Bones

The most important minerals are calcium, phosphorus, and magnesium, but without the protein matrix that's the infrastructure of bone, there would be nothing to mineralize. This underscores the importance of getting the right levels of protein every day of the week.

Dr. Katherine Tucker of Tufts University in Boston compared diets and bone density of Framingham study adults who were sixty-nine to ninety-seven, and she found that the more animal protein people ate, the higher the bone density. Other researchers reached similar conclusions when they studied younger women. This information is at odds with the popular belief that eating too much protein will cause bone loss.

Dr. Jane Kerstetter of the University of Connecticut reviewed protein intake in relation to bone metabolism and saw that the optimal protein intake for younger and older adults with respect to bone mass is between 1 and 1.5 grams per kilogram of lean body weight, or 0.45 to 0.68 gram per pound of lean body weight. Lean body weight is a BMI between 18 and 25. This is about 50 percent more than the recommendation from the Food and Nutrition Board of the National Academy of Sciences: 0.36 gram per pound per day.

Remember, though, that protein contributes to the production of acid—and vegetables and fruits that are high in potassium and magnesium act as antacids and buffer the acid created by dietary protein.

If you're shooting for the best bone production, consume more protein and fresh produce than most North Americans eat. Furthermore, maintain a 3:1 produce-to-protein ratio to keep the right acid-base balance for tamping down bone turnover.

A growing child is a construction project. Genes are the blueprints. Of all of the building blocks required to grow a human being, the most important are vegetables and protein, followed by healthy fat. Least important are carbohydrates.

A new finding suggests that in order to have healthy bones, a child needs more protein than researchers once thought was necessary. Recent studies from the Hospital for Sick Children in Toronto estimate the protein needs of children at 0.7 grams per pound of lean body weight. This amounts to about 50 percent more than adult maintenance requirements (see chapter 6).

To have room in their stomachs for the green, leafy veggies, fruits, and lean protein required for building healthy bones, most people have to dramatically reduce or eliminate their intake of pastas, cereals, breads, and cheeses.

Exercising for Bone Health

Exercise makes you a lot more likely to meet and keep your prime bone—that important peak bone mass.

Studies in children, young women, athletes, and astronauts all show that weight-bearing and resistance exercise help produce new bone. The more exercise and resistance training you do regularly, the greater your bone production and the higher your bone mass. Conversely, sedentary individuals, including those who are immobilized due to hospitalization, have dramatic increases in bone turnover and bone loss.

Rickets and Osteomalacia

If osteoporosis is bone demineralization, rickets in children and osteomalacia in adults represent the failure to mineralize new bone. A person with rickets may have bone and joint pain, deformation and bending of bones (bowlegs, knock-knees, scoliosis), widened joints, fractures, and abnormal growth rates. Osteomalacia has many symptoms, including fatigue, bone pain, joint pain/swelling, muscle pain, weakness, and a propensity to fractures.

Mineralization of new bone is the key element that goes wrong in rickets and osteomalacia. The problem can occur in either of the two stages of bone mineralization.

The primary phase, which takes weeks to months, marks the time when calcium and magnesium are added to the collagen framework. Secondary mineralization, which takes months to years, is supposed to create strong, stable bone, but high bone turnover can cut short that secondary mineralization, leaving bone that's not structurally stable. If the bone is lacking in structural stability, it can bend or warp (rickets) or be brittle and break easily (osteomalacia and osteoporosis).

Most people think of rickets and osteomalacia as vitamin D–deficiency bone diseases, but these are actually diseases caused by lack of protein, vitamin D, magnesium, and calcium. Children and adults who are protein malnourished (vegetarians) develop symptoms of these diseases at higher vitamin D levels than do people who consume adequate protein. This means that good nutrition allows you to tolerate lower vitamin D levels without suffering from bone problems.

There is a vitamin D threshold below which bone disease becomes possible. A 2010 study in Germany looked at the bone composition of healthy adults who died in accidents. They found that mineralization of bone was never abnormal in the ones who had a vitamin D level higher than 30 ng/mL. The further the D level was below this threshold, the more likely abnormal bone mineralization occurred in these people.

Good Bones, Good Teeth

Dental health when you're a child—and dental health throughout life—parallel what's happening in your bones. Your teeth—number, composition, and quality—are influenced by sufficient or insufficient protein, calcium, magnesium, and vitamin D during fetal development and early childhood. When you're an adult, these nutrients and alkaline saliva help to maintain teeth and gum health.

Albert came to see me at the Arthritis Institute because he was experiencing pain in his jaw and in many of his teeth, some loose teeth, and muscle and joint pains. After starting the Vitamin D Cure, he had great results: the pain in his teeth and jaw stopped, his joint/muscle pain resolved, and his teeth were no longer loose.

People with extensive tooth loss almost always have low vitamin D levels and low bone mass. Calcium and vitamin D supplementation, however, can reduce their rate of tooth loss. Early tooth loss and tooth/gum pain also are symptoms of inadequate bone production, accelerated bone turnover, and/or bone loss.

Many studies have revealed a link between gum disease, cavities, and/or tooth loss and the incidence of cardiovascular disease and multiple sclerosis. Gum disease is associated with the development of cardiovascular disease, even after accounting for other variables. Again, vitamin D deficiency is a common variable.

LOLA'S STORY

Lola, thirty-seven, is a good example of the health vulnerability of young mothers. Too often, people attribute fatigue and body aches to the increased demands involved in taking care of young children. In truth, the problems are the demands of pregnancy and breast-feeding on a woman's body, especially when there are pregnancies within two years. This situation often drains the nutrient stores of the mother—protein and minerals—increasing her likelihood of experiencing symptoms from low vitamin D levels.

It's not unusual to see a woman have cavities, gum disease, and loose, painful teeth in the year following childbirth/breast-feeding, which shows that a pregnant woman's body "gives" to the baby at the expense of her own stores of protein, vitamin D, and calcium.

Pregnancy and breast-feeding are stress tests for the mother because it takes enhanced nutrition and extra physical activity to maintain bone and muscle mass. With ideal vitamin D levels and improved nutrition, you can ensure the health of a mother and the fetus as the pregnancy progresses and after delivery as well.

The mother of two preschoolers, Lola had pain in her shoulders, arms, and hands when she was referred to us for evaluation because she had an elevated rheumatoid factor. Other health problems included fatigue, headaches, neck pain, mild anxiety, and depression.

She had no swollen joints, but she was experiencing muscle and bone tenderness and very sensitive shins. Generally, she was in good health. Lab studies revealed a rheumatoid factor of 20 (normal is 10 or less). All of her other studies were normal.

Her initial CLINHAQII scores were 0.375–55–15–30–6 (function, pain, fatigue, health perception, sleep). Her vitamin D level was 22; her PTH and calcium levels were normal.

We started Lola on vitamin D 30 IU per pound per day as well as some calcium and magnesium. Her diet changes were reduced salt, cheese, and grains, and an increased intake of fresh produce and lean meat at a 3:1 ratio.

Three months later, Lola had improved greatly, posting these results:

- CLINHAQII scores of 0–15–0–30–7
- Vitamin D score of 53
- Normal function
- Pain reduced by 70 percent
- Minimal fatigue

Kidney Stones

A combination of changes in urine chemistry causes kidney stones—and your vitamin D metabolism and your diet influence these changes.

About 12 percent of Americans will have a kidney stone at some point, and the incidence is growing. Between 1950 and 1974, the number of kidney stones rose from 79 cases per 100,000 adult Americans to 124 cases per 100,000 adult Americans. This incidence is also rising in countries as diverse as the Netherlands and Japan.

African Americans have a fourfold lower risk of kidney stones compared to European Americans, probably due to lower calcium excretion in the urine in response to vitamin D deficiency. Many kidney-stone formers produce more than one type of stone. African Americans have fewer stones that contain calcium and phosphorus, but they have more uric acid stones than European Americans.

The lower your vitamin D levels, the less calcium you lose in your urine. The kidneys are holding on to calcium, conserving calcium, when a person is vitamin D-deficient.

We see high PTH levels accompanying high blood pressure in both African Americans and European Americans. Higher blood pressure and PTH levels are associated with higher uric acid levels. The longer a patient has had high blood pressure, the higher the uric acid level and the greater the degree of kidney dysfunction. According to statistics, African Americans have more kidney dysfunction stemming from high blood pressure. Furthermore, a person whose kidneys aren't working well has a limited ability to handle dietary acidosis, which contributes to forming uric acid kidney stones.

Why are there more kidney stones today? The answer is urbanization of diets. The two diet elements that figure into kidney stone formation are hydration and acid-base balance, determined by dietary composition.

Calcium-containing stones are the most common, but what regulates the concentration of calcium in urine is your daily intake of water, salt, potassium, magnesium, calcium, and protein. The less water you drink, the higher the concentration of calcium and acid in your urine and the higher your risk for stone formation. Similarly, the more calcium you take in, the more you have available to discard in urine.

The NHANES study results tell us that European Americans eat more dairy than African Americans. This higher calcium intake, along with higher D levels, lead to a greater absorption of calcium and, subsequently, a higher rate of loss in the urine. African Americans, Latin Americans, and Asian Americans consume less dairy due to lactose intolerance. Combined with lower vitamin D levels, this leads to lower urine calcium losses.

A typical urban diet has a high protein-to-potassium ratio (vegetables and fruits) compared to primitive diets. Drs. Anthony Sebastian and Lynda Frasetto of the University of California at San Francisco have demonstrated that diets with a high intake of protein compared to potassium produce acidic urine. As we age and as kidney function declines, so does our ability to neutralize the acid delivered to our kidneys. Acidic urine is more likely to lead to the development of kidney stones.

The principal source of antacid to neutralize this metabolic acidosis comes from your intake of potassium, magnesium, and, to a lesser degree, calcium in the form of fresh produce. If you don't get these from your diet, you have to borrow antacid from your musculoskeletal system, where you find potassium in the muscle, and calcium and magnesium in the bone.

As your salt intake goes up, you lose more and more potassium, magnesium, and calcium in your urine. A chronic high salt intake, combined with this acidosis, leads to increased losses of these minerals in a low-volume, acidic urine. That, in turn, can make you form stones.

The key to kidney stone prevention is drinking plenty of water; balancing the acid-base in your diet; and if your vitamin D level is normal, avoiding excess calcium.

Lowering Your Risk

We estimate that the recommendations in the Vitamin D Cure will lower your risk of arthritis by about 50 percent. The risk of muscle weakness, loss of coordination, and falling associated with aging should drop by 50 percent with fortification of vitamin D. Available information on the effects of vitamin D on bone examines older adults with established disease, and they show a 26 percent reduction in the risk of osteoporosis with higher vitamin D. However, if fortification of vitamin D and diet begin during fetal development and childhood, the risk for bone and joint disease is likely to be reduced by more than 50 percent.

14

Your Most Important Health Move Ever

Legend has it that Juan Ponce de León left Puerto Rico and other Caribbean islands in search of the Fountain of Youth. As it turns out, he did discover the Fountain of Youth in the form of Florida. Florida is the Sunshine State and the southernmost point in the continental United States—and a destination for more retirees than any other state. Furthermore, it's also a major source of fresh produce from farming and seafood. UVB light is available in Florida essentially year round for the production of vitamin D.

This is significant today—even more than historically—because vitamin D and a healthy diet represent a real Fountain of Youth. The most prevalent health problems of old age are arthritis, osteoporosis, heart disease, cancer, and dementia, and all of these respond favorably to normalization of vitamin D levels and diet.

The Vitamin D Cure goes beyond the mythical Fountain of Youth for seniors because it's a Fountain *for* Youth, too. Adequate vitamin D and an acid-base-balanced diet in the developing fetus and in growing children will:

- ensure healthy brain development;
- reduce risk of infection;
- improve response to vaccines;
- build stronger bones and teeth;
- reduce the risk of arthritis, scoliosis, high blood pressure, diabetes, heart disease, and autoimmune diseases in later life; and
- reduce the risk of breast cancer, prostate cancer, and other malignancies in later life.

You can accumulate all of this protection before puberty ends!

This book empowers a new century of readers to see past traditional thinking and invest in the new science, simplicity, and success of lifestyle changes that can restore your body chemistry and grant you better health for the rest of your life.

The Big Picture

What I now know about health connections to vitamin D deficiency and diet has radically changed the way I view patient problems. All health problems are connected. A person's high blood pressure and diabetes are now part of the same disease that's causing his arthritis and bone disease. I no longer pigeonhole symptoms into separate diagnoses and then address only the ones I know well.

You could say I'm a physician who has renewed interest in the total patient. If someone has a family history of diabetes, high blood pressure, and heart disease, she gets an automatic assessment for risks of vitamin D deficiency and dietary imbalance. Histories of infections or malignancy, breast-feeding, dental problems, kidney stones, and childhood residences are now relevant pieces of the puzzle.

I make it clear to my patients that all of their problems are connected and that they have control over their health. After fixing their vitamin D and diet deficiencies, many people report dramatic changes in the way they feel. Not only do they eliminate all the pain they've been suffering for years, they're also losing weight and lowering their blood pressure. Everyone is shocked by the simplicity of the solution.

To be sure, addressing vitamin D and diet deficiencies isn't a cure-all, and you may not be able to throw away all of your meds for a bottle of vitamin D. But you can use the ideas in this book to complement other therapies. You can reduce your dependence on medications because your symptoms will be eased or erased. The benefits of the therapies you've been using will be enhanced by vitamin D supplementation and a better diet.

In today's high-tech, urbanized society, vitamin D deficiency, dietary imbalances, and couch potato-ness are enormous bottlenecks in the quest for health. But the impact of correcting vitamin D and dietary deficiencies on your health will be more profound and less costly than any other interventions you could try.

A healthy lifestyle can even drown out genetic differences. Genetics then becomes background noise that's irrelevant. You'll find that your health isn't in your genes any more than it's something projected on you by outside pressures.

Your genes are a collection of notes, almost exactly the same notes we're all given. What's different is the music you make with them, and that determines your health and happiness. Why not select health and happiness over history and habit by taking the route that will give you a more fulfilling life—the Vitamin D Cure?

If the image you have of yourself is fat, tired, and hurting, that will be your reality. But if you change your internal image, you'll find that it's easier to make the choices necessary to bring that new and improved image to life.

A key element of the entire process is reframing what you think about yourself. The most common complaint I hear when I suggest a target weight to patients is "Oh, I haven't weighed that little since high school!" All that means is that this individual doesn't expect to hit that low weight ever again. She's subscribing to the theory that time takes its toll; she's just a victim of the ravages of years.

Another patient will say "Diabetes runs in the family," meaning that his genetics predetermines his fate. He *will* have diabetes at some point, he assures himself, and he has always expected that the day of doom would come.

But let the evidence in this book convince you otherwise. Health isn't about genes, it's about choices.

Capture a healthy image in your mind, massage that idea, and shoot for your best goal with all your energy and optimism. Make a list of foods and go grocery shopping to restock your shelves. Figure out the dose of vitamin D you need and get started right away on your supplementation. Start moving! Don't make it complicated.

Eat better. Pump up your vitamin D levels. Within ninety days you'll be feeling better and your only question will be *Why didn't I make these changes years ago?*

Go to www.thevitamindcure.com for the latest information on vitamin D and dietary acid-base balance.

Vitamin D Cure
Questions and Answers

Q: The latest report on vitamin D and calcium from the Institute of Medicine says that most Americans get enough vitamin D and don't need supplements. So why do you say we all are deficient and need supplements?

A: The Institute of Medicine (www.IOM.edu) revised its vitamin D and calcium recommendations in late 2010. The institute increased the DRI-RDA for vitamin D from 400 IU to 600 IU and raised the maximum safe daily intake of vitamin D to 4,000 IU. The Institute's recommendations for calcium are complicated because they are different for infants, children, adults, and older adults. Although these changes move in the right direction, they fall short of the recommendations published by panels of vitamin D researchers, and they fail to meet public health needs.

In contrast, a panel of twenty-five world experts in vitamin D research convened in Paris in late 2009 for a Vitamin D Summit. The goal of the meeting was to answer four questions. Who should be tested for vitamin D deficiency? What is a normal vitamin D level? Who should be supplemented? And when should testing be done? After an extensive review of the literature, the panel recommended testing all people with or at risk for developing autoimmune disease, muscle and bone disease, heart disease, and cancer. The panel also concluded that a normal D level is between 30 and 100 ng/mL (75–250 nmol/L). In addition, the committee agreed that those with vitamin D deficiency or dark skin, as well as institutionalized people, should be supplemented starting at 800 IU and the amount increased as needed to raise the blood level into the normal range. Finally, the committee members suggested that monitoring shouldn't start until at least three months after beginning supplementation. All of these guidelines are consistent with the recommendations of this book. For a more detailed answer and links to the science, see the archives of the *Vitamin D Blog* at www.thevitamindcure.com.

$Q:$ What is the difference between vitamin D_2 and vitamin D_3? Which one should I take?

$A:$ There are two forms of vitamin D: vitamin D_2 (ergocalciferol or Drisdol, the prescription form of D_2) and D_3 (cholecalciferol, which is not prescribed in the United States but is available without prescription). Vitamin D_2 comes from plants. Mammals make D_3 from cholesterol with the assistance of UVB radiation and heat. You metabolize a dose of vitamin D_2 by half in about seven days, with complete elimination in two weeks. You metabolize a dose of vitamin D_3 by half in about 10 weeks. Peak blood levels of vitamin D_2 are 30 percent lower than D_3 after the same dose.

  1,000 IU D3 = 1,300 IU D_2, if dosed daily
  1,000 IU D3 = 4,000 IU D_2, if dosed weekly

You must take vitamin D_2 at least twice a week, or preferably daily, to adjust for rapid elimination and lower peak levels. In general, weekly or monthly dosing of D_2 won't produce significant rises in vitamin D levels or vitamin D effects.

A recent review on the effects of vitamin D on bone confirms the inefficacy of vitamin D_2 as it is commonly prescribed. Unfortunately, there is only one dose of D_2 readily available in the United States, and this is a 50,000 IU gel cap. That is like trying to do eye surgery with a butter knife—you're using the wrong tool for the job.

Touting vitamin D_2 products, several small manufacturers cater to vegetarians, but vegetarians should take into account these dosing differences and also verify the purity of the products they buy.

Vitamin D_3 replacement at a given dose reaches steady state in ten weeks. The long half-life of vitamin D_3 allows for missed doses without a significant drop in blood level. It also allows for makeup doses and weekly or monthly dosing, while still maintaining a steady blood level.

You can buy over-the-counter vitamin D_3 at a very low cost. A year's supply of vitamin D_3 gel caps costs less than $20. The co-pay for prescription vitamin D_2 is as much as a month's supply of D_3. So for prescription vitamin D_2—those little green gel caps—you end up paying eight to ten times as much for about three to four times less effective vitamin D, based on weekly dosing.

Q: Isn't fifteen minutes of casual sun exposure daily enough to make all of the vitamin D I need?

A: First, look at that fifteen minutes. You have to be getting sun during the right season—when ultraviolet B light is available. This usually means late spring, summer, and early fall. Next, you need to be exposed to sun intense enough to make vitamin D in only fifteen minutes. Usually, that intensity is available in only mid-summer (UV index of 7). Next, you must have enough skin exposed, as solar panels would be, to alter the vitamin D in your skin. This means 50 percent or more of your skin surface has to get sunrays. You can meet these requirements more easily in Florida, Texas, Southern California, and Hawaii. In other states, this opportunity is limited to the summertime. In other words, you have to wear your swimsuit under your work clothes for lunch-break sun exposure in the summer.

Q: Your book recommends limiting calcium to no more than 600 mg a day. Other doctors and news reports say that I should take 1,200 to 1,500 mg a day. Why is your recommendation so different? I was under the impression I needed calcium for aging bones.

A: Your calcium needs drop when you normalize your vitamin D levels because of the increased absorption of calcium from your diet (see chapter 7). Published in late 2007, a review of studies on the use of calcium supplements to protect bone showed that calcium alone doesn't prevent fractures. Worse, a 2010 review in the *British Medical Journal* suggests that supplementing with calcium in the absence of vitamin D may result in an increased risk of having a heart attack and possibly a stroke. Calcium supplements may also increase your risk of developing kidney stones and prostate cancer.

Plus, there are other reasons you don't need a great deal of supplemental calcium or dairy. Wild animals don't supplement calcium, and they don't have weak bones and teeth. A wild elephant gets all of the calcium it needs for its large bones and teeth from vegetables, which make up its entire diet.

The message is this: Focus on getting your calcium from lots of green leafy vegetables. Take vitamin D supplements, exercise, and steer clear of calcium supplements and dairy products.

Q: What are the latest vitamin D recommendations?

A: In June 2011, the Endocrine Society published clinical practice guidelines for vitamin D–deficiency screening and treatment. The committee chair was Dr. Michael Holick. Members included calcium/vitamin D experts Drs. Robert Heaney, Neil Binkley, and Heike Bischoff-Ferrari. The guidelines recommended were:

- Measure vitamin D in all people who are at risk for deficiency. (*The Vitamin D Cure* recommends screening the general population for vitamin D deficiency.)
- Take vitamin D supplements to achieve a consistent blood level higher than 30 ng/mL. (A level of 40 ng/mL is ideal.)

These guidelines agree with the recommendations you will find in this book.

Although committee recommendations suggest different amounts of vitamin D for various age groups, you can follow weight-based dosing and eliminate age considerations. Note: Vitamin D_2 for replacement isn't a good idea, due to its high cost and the body's rapid metabolism of D_2.

Q: Do some medications interfere with vitamin D absorption or action?

A: Any medication that reduces cholesterol absorption from the gut will also reduce vitamin D absorption. This includes bile acid–binding agents such as cholestyramine (Questran, Colestid). New medications that may lower vitamin D absorption are ezetimibe (Zetia, Vytorin).

Even when using vitamin D supplements, many people who take these medications cannot elevate their vitamin D levels. In some cases, they avoid problems by taking vitamin D twelve hours before or after the medications. If you take any of the meds listed previously, make sure you have your vitamin D level tested.

Other problematic drugs insofar as keeping your vitamin D level high enough are anticonvulsants, including diphenylhydantoin or phenytoin (Dilantin), carbamazepine (Tegretol), phenobarbital (Luminal), oxcarbazepine (Trileptal), clonazepam (Klonipin), and valproate (Depakote, Depakene).

Phenytoin, carbamazepine, and phenobarbital activate the enzymes that break down vitamin D, thus reducing its activity. These drugs may also interfere with parathyroid hormone action, calcitonin (calcium-regulating hormones), and calcium absorption. Some of the drugs also impede steroid hormone metabolism, by lowering effective androgen and estrogen levels, which adversely affects bone turnover.

Doctors should screen people for vitamin D deficiency if they take anticonvulsants, should recommend vitamin D supplements, and should monitor compliance. This is especially important in the case of children who are on anticonvulsants.

It is interesting to note that vitamin D has anticonvulsant properties in both animals and humans. People may be able to reduce their risk of having seizures by taking D supplements and by increasing their intake of foods with omega-3 fats and magnesium.

Q: Since I had gastric bypass surgery, I have had great difficulty in getting my vitamin D level back to normal? Why?

A: Traditional gastric bypass surgery often removes more than 90 percent of the stomach. It bypasses the early small bowel, referred to as the duodenum, and in a modified procedure can bypass much of the small bowel, causing defective absorption of minerals, vitamin B_{12}, fat, and fat-soluble nutrients such as vitamin D. Many obese people simply don't take enough supplemental vitamin D to normalize their levels based on their weight. After gastric bypass, however, they also may not be absorbing the vitamin D for several reasons. First, if most of the small bowel was bypassed, then the portion that absorbs fat and fat-soluble vitamins is not seeing any food. This causes these people to have a flawed ability to absorb essential fatty acids, including omega-3 fats and vitamins A, D, E, and K.

You get vitamin A from a normal diet, and your requirements of vitamins E and K are minimal. Vitamin D and omega-3 are the crucial missing nutrients that require supplementation. Second, if a doctor removes or bypasses too much of the small bowel, as in surgery for inflammatory bowel disease, the patient may experience chronic diarrhea, which further reduces the absorption of all nutrients (protein, fat, carbohydrates) due to the very rapid transit of food through the gut.

The challenge of obtaining adequate nutrition in gastric bypass or bowel surgery patients is to overcome the decreased amount of bowel available for absorption. Pureed foods enhance the absorption of macronutrients and minerals. Eating small, frequent meals can require less surface area for absorption. High-quality foods (lean meats and green veggies) are necessary to fit the most nutrition into the smallest packages. This is the paradox of gastric bypass surgery, which many people undergo to avoid making lifestyle changes. Ultimately, the patient needs to change what and how much he or she eats.

In people whose vitamin D levels don't normalize with standard dosing (see chapter 5), taking more vitamin D usually doesn't work. But light therapy may serve to normalize their vitamin D. You can use a vitamin D (UVB) lamp at home or you can try tanning bed UVB therapy. Sperti Ultraviolet Systems (www.sperti.com) sells personal vitamin D UVB lamps.

Tanning beds expose users to large amounts of UVA, which may be more harmful than UVB. Many dermatologists and other doctors offer narrow-band UVB light therapy.

Q: I have seen blood spot tests available online to measure vitamin D levels. Are these tests accurate?

A: Several companies manufacture blood spot tests for vitamin D. You mail your sample to a central lab, where it is analyzed with liquid chromatography and mass spectroscopy. These tests can be as accurate at measuring vitamin D from drawn blood. ZRT Labs (www.zrtlab.com) offers the most widely available and reliable tests. You can buy these tests online, but they may not be reimbursed by your insurance. Health insurance usually does, however, cover traditional blood level testing in your doctor's office.

Q: I noticed that the Vitamin D Cure discourages dairy. This makes me wonder what's appropriate for children. Pediatricians recommend that children two or younger drink whole milk, and you mention only low-fat. What's the story? Also, what about cheese for kids?

A: Dairy isn't as healthy as lean meat and vegetables because of the sugar factor. The lactose in milk is a simple sugar. Milk is a complete nutritional package for children younger than one, but it also provides excess sugar that they *don't* need after the first year of life. The combo of simple sugar and protein promotes insulin resistance.

Protein is a more potent stimulus for insulin release than sugar; the combination of protein and sugar shoots your insulin *way up*, causing insulin resistance. That's why you are better off with lean protein and vegetables. Unsalted natural nut butter is a better choice than cheese— it has just as much protein but healthier fat and no salt.

Feed fish and chicken to children one and older. Remember that your child's metabolism is still trying to find its set point in the first few years of life—and he's developing tastes, so you don't want to send the wrong signals to his metabolism and taste buds.

Remember, too, that most recommendations for children's milk intake are faulty. All of the fat in whole milk is saturated, which is no better for your health at six months of age than it is at six or sixty. About 84 percent of whole milk calories come from sugar and saturated fat. And no one wants to stuff her kids with sugar and saturated fat.

A child older than one who drinks whole milk gets too much saturated fat and sugar, which feeds the wrong bacteria in the intestines at a vulnerable age. Whole milk is not an ideal food; only 16 percent of its calories are protein, and that's no better than eating bread.

Kids need polyunsaturated fat—both omega-6 and omega-3 fat—in a ratio of 5:1 or less. You can ensure that your children get this all-important balance of polyunsaturated fats via:

- Fish oil supplements
- Omega-3 supplements
- Canola oil
- Flax oil
- Walnut butter or another natural, unsalted nut butter
- Green vegetables

Q: I've always heard that white cheese is healthier than yellow. Is this correct?

A: No, both white and yellow are high-fat and contain the wrong kind of fat. Both have lots of salt and many calories. Neither contributes to good health. Typically, cheeses that are softer and have more moisture, such as cottage cheese, feta cheese, and goat cheese, are less acidic. Their acid content is on a par with a serving of meat, but their nutritional value still lags—less protein, more fat, and more salt.

Q: I was a beach kid, getting lots of sun for the first twenty years of my life. Does my vitamin D "heritage" help me now that I'm fifty? I know my skin took a toll from the sun; I have lots of brown spots and skin tags.

A: People think they store vitamin D, but this isn't true. You don't store vitamins—or, in this case, a hormone. All bioactive nutrients have a half-life—that's how long the substance is in your body before half of it is used up. Some nutrients, such as vitamin C, have very short half-lives. Vitamin C is half gone in 30 minutes. Vitamin D is a hormone system that has numerous variations or metabolites, all with varying degrees of activity and importance. This book focuses on two of these, but there are many more. Because it's not really one molecule, we can't measure its half-life precisely because it varies, depending on which one you're measuring and the situation you're measuring it in.

The vitamin D measured in blood tests (25 hydroxy vitamin D_3) has about a two-and-a-half-month half-life, meaning that half of it is gone in two to three months. This form of vitamin D is a reflection of your sun exposure, diet, and activity level.

Your question refers to lasting benefit. Benefit does carry over, especially if your vitamin D levels were normal (50 to 70) during the first twenty years of your life. Normal vitamin D levels in childhood ensure development of a healthy immune system, and that lowers your risk of immune-mediated diseases later in life, such as thyroid disease, multiple sclerosis, type 1 diabetes, lupus, and rheumatoid arthritis. A healthy immune system also helps you fight or prevent cancer. Normal vitamin D levels during your childhood build more bone so that you are more likely to reach peak bone mass. Reaching optimal bone mass lowers your risk of fractures for life. Normal vitamin D levels while you were in your mother's womb reduce your risk for obesity, hypertension, diabetes, cholesterol problems, and nervous system diseases. Vitamin D is extremely important in the first twenty years of your life because it may ensure health in the last twenty.

Q: I read that we get more colds and flu in the winter because we don't get enough vitamin D then—less UV light due to the sun's angle in the winter sky and the fact that we're bundled up in coats. Is this true?

A: This is true. More respiratory infections during winter are probably directly related to lower vitamin D production. Several factors increase your likelihood of catching an infection in the winter. Ultraviolet light in the "B" spectrum inactivates many viruses, so that means that in the summer, viruses don't survive outside your body as long as they do in the winter, when there is less UVB getting through the ozone. D levels begin to fall in the fall. When the leaves start turning colors, the amount of UVB available to make vitamin D is negligible. In Michigan, for example, that's usually mid- or late September. By Thanksgiving and Christmas, in the upper half of the United States, many people have very low D levels. Worldwide, the same phenomenon occurs, moving from the Northern to the Southern Hemisphere as the seasons change, and the wave of respiratory illnesses (including flu) follows. Vitamin D turns out to be very important in your immune system's defense against viral and bacterial attack. As less vitamin D is available, your immune system's ability to mobilize the right cells in the right places becomes sluggish. Your immune system is also less able to produce antimicrobial proteins that kill bacteria. As a result, respiratory infection rates typically begin to rise in late September and peak in about February.

In winter you should forget chicken soup with lots of noodles and salt and too little chicken and instead take your vitamin D, vacation in the sun in December and again in February if you can, and eat healthy.

Q: What can I eat at a picnic if candy, hot dogs, nachos, and popcorn are all forbidden on this diet? And what about barbecue sandwiches, coleslaw, beer, and chips? Do you have some alternatives that people can manage?

A: Some of my favorite foods are barbecued spareribs and cornbread with butter, corn chips with salsa, chocolate, commercial peanut butter, and old-fashioned chili made of red meat. But these also give me indigestion, gas, and heartburn. I look for ways to make my favorite foods healthier. You may want to try the following ideas:

- Make barbecued spareribs *without* gobs of commercial sauce loaded with salt, sugar, butter, and vinegar; instead, use a spicy sauce of pineapple juice, citrus, and chili pepper.

- Replace corn chips with sweet potato chips or taro chips cooked in expeller-pressed canola oil with very little sodium.

- Choose dark chocolate over milk chocolate. And eat less.

- Eat natural, unsalted nut butter instead of commercial nut butter. Try almond butter.

- Make chili with lean, ground round (or turkey breast), fewer beans, and no-salt-added canned tomatoes. Top with cilantro and guacamole instead of cheese.

Unfortunately, some foods are impossible to "healthy up." Examples are processed meats such as hot dogs and cheese dips. Eat these bad boys no more than two or three times a year: July Fourth, the Super Bowl, and a free pass.

Just because a meal is an old family favorite doesn't make it great for your health.

Q: Why do so many people in industrialized countries have D deficiencies when these people have better access to good foods?

A: The simple answer is that vitamin D usually doesn't come from food. We make it when we're exposed to sunshine. Only about 10 percent of your vitamin D comes from diet. In fact, the more technologically advanced a nation becomes, the less time people spend outdoors at midday and the more time they spend indoors behind machines or computers.

Why are rickets and severe D deficiency so common in poor and unindustrialized countries? The answer is that many of these countries are poverty-ridden, and when you're malnourished in protein and fat, that reduces your production of cholesterol, which is the precursor to vitamin D. If your liver doesn't have the protein or fat required to make cholesterol, you can't make pre-vitamin D, which is what you need so that sun rays can convert D to usable vitamin D.

Q: How does the impact of vitamin D supplementation compare to the effect of a drug, such as an antibiotic?

A: Vitamin D has many complex effects on immune response to infection, unlike an antibiotic, which generally inhibits a single enzyme or interferes with one aspect of cellular function. The beauty of a normal vitamin D level is that it's likely to prevent your need for antibiotics by avoiding serious infection altogether. In the case of an infection, your adequate vitamin D level should speed clearance of the microbe and reduce the likelihood of incomplete eradication of the microbe or the development of antibiotic resistance. The vitamin D and the antibiotic team up to overcome infection more quickly and completely. Moreover, vitamin D will assist in the repair of damaged tissues after an infection, too. Vitamin D speeds wound healing, and antibiotics in the absence of a functioning immune system aren't effective. We see this all the time in bone marrow transplant patients and cancer patients who are undergoing chemotherapy. In the end, it is not about either/or—it's about teamwork. Simply put, vitamin D can help antibiotics work better.

Q: If I eat well 80 percent of the time, is that enough to correct my acid-base imbalance?

A: Certainly, 80 percent is better than something less. That means you're eating four meals a week that don't comply with the recommendations. Better to have only one or two meals per week that fall off the wagon. When my patients say they are doing the diet 80 percent of the time, this can mean different things to different people. Essentially, though, 80 percent means that eight of ten meals are on the plan. You should bank extra vegetables and fruits and protein; that way, even if you abandon the food plan 20 percent of the time by eating grain, cheese, and salt, it won't be hard to bring yourself back to acid-base balance. But remember those bacteria in your gut—they may not respond as quickly to these swings in your diet. Exercise and supplementation also can buy you some diet leeway.

Q: What if I do all of the things you recommend except the exercise component?

A: Exercise is an important part of the regimen. Though you may lose weight and feel better by making dietary changes, all of these improvements are supercharged when you add exercise to your routine. Exercising before meals doubles the benefit of your workout by reducing the amount you eat and by increasing your metabolic rate in the period after your meal. Exercise triggers growth hormone release, driving good nutrition into your bones and muscles. You will also find that exercise helps your mood and the quality of your sleep. Plus, doing workouts gives you some wiggle room with your diet. So, don't undercut your program benefits by leaving out exercise.

Q: What are the best vitamin D–rich foods?

A: You get the most vitamin D from cold-water fish that are high in omega-3 fatty acids—herring, salmon, halibut, wild channel catfish, mackerel, tuna, and sardines—fish that contain 250 to 650 IU per 3.5-ounce serving. Fresh fish has more D than canned, and raw fish has more than cooked. One source of large amounts of vitamin D_2 is dried shiitake mushrooms, which have 1,660 IU per 3.5-ounce serving. Dole Foods takes this up a notch by pulsing its shiitake mushrooms with ultraviolet B light to enhance the vitamin D content. All milk, regardless of fat content, has 100 IU of vitamin D per 8-ounce glass. You also can buy orange juice with that same amount of D per glass. An egg yolk is another good source (100 IU of D in one egg).

Q: If the immune system is largely formed during fetal growth and childhood, can doing the right things in adulthood really alter basic immune system deficits that were set up early in life?

A: If you already have type 1 diabetes or multiple sclerosis, taking vitamin D won't cure your disease. This is true of all autoimmune diseases that have a vitamin D deficiency connection. The events that triggered your diabetes or MS are history that you can't change. However, you can improve glucose control, insulin sensitivity, and probably the frequency and intensity of MS attacks by correcting vitamin D after you develop the disease. In other words, optimizing vitamin D and diet will reduce your disease activity and/or slow progression of your disease.

You can enhance the effects of vitamin D and diet on your immune system's response to infection and aspects of cancer surveillance at any point in your life by improving your vitamin D levels and diet.

Q: Some people take cod-liver oil for its D content, but it tastes awful and leaves an aftertaste. Is there a more palatable way to take it? What about fish oil tablets or pills?

A: A teaspoon of cod-liver oil has 450 IU of vitamin D and 4,500 IU of vitamin A. It also has about 850 milligrams of omega-3 fatty acid. Taking cod-liver oil in gelcaps eliminates having to taste it, but you still may have reflux symptoms and belching. Gelcaps are best because they reduce the likelihood of oxidation, which causes unstable fats such as omega-3 fat to go rancid. Adults aren't good candidates for taking cod-liver oil as a vitamin D supplement simply because they will get too much vitamin A. A teaspoon of cod-liver oil slightly exceeds the DRI for vitamin A in adults.

Q: How do you rate the nutrition value of sardines, tuna, and low-fat and no-fat cottage cheese and yogurt?

A: Canned sardines and tuna are excellent sources of protein and omega-3 fatty acids, and sardines have about 500 IU of vitamin D per 3.75-ounce can, with tuna providing about half as much vitamin D. Cottage cheese is a soft cheese that produces less acid than processed cheese or cheddar cheese. The acid value of cottage cheese is about 9 for a 3.5-ounce serving, similar to that for tuna. Cottage cheese has half as much protein as an equivalent serving of lean meat, and depending on fat content, may have more or less fat. Yogurt has half as much protein as cottage cheese per equivalent serving and typically more grams of carbs than cottage cheese or meat due to sweeteners and fruit added for taste. Unless they are nonfat products, the dairy products have saturated fat but no omega-3 fat. Tuna has about 30 more calories in a 3.5-ounce serving than the dairy, but this is a situation that calls for choosing nutrients without worrying about calories. Fish is better than dairy.

Q: If it's really as simple as two main food groups (protein and produce) for good health, why do so many nutritionists and doctors recommend cheese as part of a healthy diet?

A: The Dairy Council has sponsored a great deal of research on dairy products in health and disease, and it's mainly this industry-sponsored research that has stimulated more research to clarify or confirm their results. For example, the DASH diet showed that adding low-fat dairy to the diet lowers blood pressure further than without dairy, especially in African Americans. This kind of research has influenced public health policy, so we get a recommendation of three servings of low-fat dairy a day—and it's now part of the USDA's "My Plate" program. The issues that haven't been addressed are: Why are three-fourths of the world's populations lactose intolerant, and how are North Americans supposed to comply with this recommendation? Would this dairy benefit evaporate if people normalized their vitamin D levels?

We're the only animals on the planet who consume other animals' breastmilk as adults. Milk is baby food designed by nature exclusively for babies. North Americans and Europeans do this either because they simply like dairy products or because milk is a cheap source of nutrition. Many people are lactose intolerant because they weren't designed to drink milk or consume dairy as adults. That means milk shouldn't be essential to your diet. You wouldn't need dairy at all if you normalized your vitamin D levels and ate more green vegetables.

Q: What about the kinds of cheese made from 2 percent milk and the low-fat versions?

A: The problems with cheese are that it's high in salt, saturated fat, and acid, and that it contains lactose. When you compare cheese to lean meat, it's just a bad source of protein. But the biggest problems with cheese are that you get burned by its acid production and you get loads of fat. Except for cottage cheese, other commonly consumed cheeses—cheddar, processed cheese, and mozzarella—produce two to three times as much acid as lean meat per equivalent serving. In general, 80 percent of the calories in a serving of cheese comes from saturated fat. When you look at the amount of cheese that average Americans consume, the numbers get scary. We put cheese on everything! In Mediterranean countries, cheese is used primarily as a garnish, like a spice—people decorate a dish with a few shavings of cheese, not globs and chunks of it. Cheese should never be your whole meal, nor should you let it be your sole protein source for a meal. Use cheese sparingly or not at all.

Q: We get salt inadvertently when we eat out and in foods we buy at the grocery store and cook at home, so how can anyone actually pull off the no-salt part of the Vitamin D Cure?

A: You can't manage a no-salt diet, and you shouldn't have a zero-sodium diet because you would die from it. But here's the rub. If I ask people about their salt intake, most say they don't add salt to their food or to dishes when they cook. But these same people eat at restaurants three to four nights a week. Because most restaurants serve you about twice the amount of food you can eat, this turns into six to eight meals a week that are probably loaded with salt. To reduce your salt intake, you have to actively avoid the stuff. Read food labels and choose the products with the least amount of salt. Factor in the times you'll be eating out and in others' homes, because that's when you just can't control salt intake. Those slips will more than make up for your personal no-salt habits.

Q: Can you recommend good breakfast foods for people who won't eat last night's leftovers?

A: Create your own new script for breakfast, and start slowly. Eggs and potatoes are okay, so you can have eggs that are scrambled, soft-boiled, hard-boiled, or poached. The cholesterol is really a nonissue. If you're concerned, get omega eggs or discard some yolks. Egg whites are pure protein and produce less acid than the whole egg. Potatoes are vegetables that are starchy and have a high glycemic index, but they're healthy compared to traditional grain breakfasts. Try sweet potatoes instead. If you want more variety, add a healthy kind of meat. Gourmet breakfasts often contain lox or salmon, but if that's too strong for you, eat a lean cut of pork, such as pork tenderloin, and fruits and vegetables.

Another option many people do not consider is skipping breakfast. If you don't get hungry until midday, you don't have to eat breakfast just because you think you should.

Most Americans are overweight or obese. No one can eat his or her way to being skinny. You have to eat fewer calories, eat healthier, and exercise.

Q: How can we become more "immuno-competent" after age forty?

A: You can make your immune system work better by following the Vitamin D Cure. Immuno-competent is just a fancy term for a healthy immune system. We know vitamin D is important early in your immune system's development, establishing tolerance to your own ecosystem yet preparing your body for microbial threats. Once your immune system becomes self-tolerant, it remains important lifelong for its protection from infection. As time goes by, the tolerance that was set up during your childhood is used as intolerance to cancer cells. Some of your ability to fight cancer later in life is probably "learned" before adolescence. To be immuno-competent, you need normal calcium and magnesium balance and adequate protein from your diet. Healthy fats, such as omega-3 fats, help reduce inflammatory substances so your immune system is quiet but ready. Finally, make sure you and your children get recommended vaccinations, which help to teach your immune system.

Q: What's the best time of day to take vitamin supplements?

A: Your body absorbs vitamins and minerals best with a meal. Protein, carbs, and fats all enhance vitamin, calcium, and magnesium absorption. Nutrients come from food, so they're best absorbed with food. Let your physician know that you're supplementing because some mineral supplements can interfere with the absorption of osteoporosis drugs, thyroid replacement, and antibiotics.

Q: Will I lose weight on the Vitamin D Cure?

A: You will lose weight if you embrace the entire program. One small study shows that supplemental vitamin D and calcium at breakfast decreases calorie intake throughout the day, but exercise is a better appetite suppressant. Normalizing vitamin D alone probably won't lead to weight loss, but it may improve your mood and energy level, spurring you to exercise. If you follow the Vitamin D Cure diet plan— the elimination of salt, cheese, and grains, combined with thirty to sixty minutes of exercise per day—weight loss is likely.

Q: I don't understand how the right diet and vitamin D levels can help me ward off cancer. Everyone in my family has had cancer of some kind, so I figure I have the genetics and it's just a matter of time. Tell me the best way to find out what I can do, or if it will make a difference.

A: Vitamin D slows the cell life cycle down. Cells grow, replicate their DNA, then divide and start the cycle over again. By slowing the life cycle, you get fewer mistakes in DNA replication. It's like slowing down an assembly line to prevent mistakes. The more mistakes that are made, the more likely a cell will transform into a cancer cell. In addition, slowing things down allows factors that promote normal differentiation and specialization to assert their effects on a cell. In this way, your cells develop appropriately. Vitamin D also turns on tumor-suppressor genes—genes that suppress the growth of cancer cells through a multi-tude of pathways, some of which also slow cell cycle. Vitamin D can facilitate cancer cell death through apoptosis, which resembles in effect the self-destructing tape on the old TV series *Mission Impossible*. And vitamin D can reduce blood flow to tumors, thus limiting their growth.

Vitamin D deficiency can affect early development of breast tissue, predisposing you to breast cancer. The same may be true for prostate cancer. Because lifestyle during childhood may be the risk factor that you and your brothers and sisters all shared, it may seem like genetics is the cause, but that's probably not true. Inherited genetics unaffected by environment accounts for less than 5 percent of cancers.

Q: I eat a good diet and take vitamins, yet I feel tired all the time, even when I first wake in the morning. I date a man who's seven years older than I am, but he has ten times more energy. How can I adjust my diet and vitamin D so I have more energy?

A: A dominant symptom of vitamin D deficiency is fatigue. The amount of vitamin D in a daily vitamin (400 IU) is typically not enough to normalize your blood level. Following the guidelines for replacement in chapter 5 may give you more energy. Another factor associated with fatigue is failure to eat enough protein. Your heart, lungs, kidneys, and brain need protein to function, and when you lack adequate protein, you borrow from your muscles and bones. If you also have an acid-base imbalance in your diet that is stealing your reserve, you're basically running on empty.

Q: My five-year-old often tells me he's "so tired." I don't understand how he can be tired because he gets enough sleep. But he's a very picky eater. Many days he eats very little, but he mainly consumes only diluted apple juice, milk, cheese, fresh fruit, carrots, chicken, turkey patties or slices, whole-wheat bread, bridge mix (pretzels and nuts), and cookies. He gets lots of sun with daily trips to the park—at least two hours per day in the sunshine (of Southern California). What's the problem?

A: At his age and living in the Southern California sun, it's unlikely that he's vitamin D-deficient. So his diet may be the problem. Most children eat too much grain and cheese, which produces acid loads that can adversely affect bone mass and behavior. Grains aren't good sources of magnesium, calcium, or potassium, and they're loaded with refined carbohydrates, which send the wrong signal to his metabolism. Protein from cheese and chicken contains only saturated fat. Forty percent of the fat in your brain is DHA, the omega-3 fat that speeds transmission of signals and probably shapes the transmission of signals. DHA binds to a vitamin A receptor along with vitamin D and goes into the nucleus of cells, where it decides which genes in the brain to turn on and which ones to turn off. Protein from lean meat (especially fresh, wild-caught fish high in omega-3 fats) and minerals from vegetables are even more critical for a developing brain than for an adult brain because children are building new structures and shaping relationships among parts of the brain. So it's key to feed children premium fuel every day.

Q: What do you think about tanning bed rays?

A: The light sources vary from place to place and from booth to booth, which makes tanning beds unpredictable and sometimes risky. Artificial UV light sources often have all three wavelengths (UVA, B, and C), and there is no ozone between you and the lightbulb. Some lights have a mixture of UVA, UVB, and no UVC that resembles sun exposure on earth. Most booths produce all three—or just lots of UVA, because it tans faster. UVC rays are dangerous to your skin and immune system. A higher ratio of UVA to UVB than the sun may be important in increasing the risk of melanoma. Overexposure to any of these wavelengths isn't healthy.

The benefits are that tanning can normalize vitamin D levels, and normal vitamin D levels reduce your risk of all cancers, including melanoma. Judicious use of artificial UV light is used to treat some skin diseases, and it can help prevent sunburns. The science is still out on whether the benefits outweigh the risks, and we really don't know what balance of UV spectrums is safest.

Q: Do people need to wear hats when they're in the sun for extended periods of time?

A: The pendulum has swung too far in the direction of sun avoidance. Our lifestyles already afford us too little sun exposure. Most of us need all the sun we can get. Estimates are that 60 to 70 percent of Americans are vitamin D–deficient, so it makes no sense to tell everyone to cover up. What is a good idea is to take care and follow the sun-exposure guidelines in chapter 5. That way you won't burn, but you will produce some vitamin D—and that's the goal.

Q: For children ages two to six, what SPF-number sunscreen or block is appropriate for a day at the beach?

A: SPF 8 (applied correctly) blocks more than 95 percent of UVB rays. SPF 15 approaches 100 percent. Depending on skin type, time of day, and season of the year, using SPF 15 should provide adequate protection if applied as stated on the label and after adequate vitamin D is made. See the tables in chapter 5 that use the UV index as a tool to help you calculate your safe sun limits. Children with extra skin melanin will tolerate longer exposure times before they need to cover up. There should be no difference in the SPF strength used to protect dark-skinned children; SPF 15 is adequate. Clothing can also be used as a sun block enabling you to avoid putting chemicals on your skin. See www.thevitamindcure.com for information on a new rating system for UVA protection.

In June 2011, the FDA announced new sunscreen labeling. It kept the familiar SPF rating for UVB protection but added "broad spectrum" to the labeling of sunscreens that also provide adequate coverage for UVA light. This means that broad-spectrum SPF 15 and higher sunscreens give you both UVA and UVB protection, which lowers your risk of skin damage/aging, as well as skin cancer. In contrast, non-broad-spectrum sunscreens and broad-spectrum sunscreens with an SPF of 2 to 14 ward off only sunburn.

Q: How can I tell if my child is getting enough sun and vitamin D?

A: Children usually don't complain of pain, fatigue, or poor sleep, so pay attention to their behavior and ask questions. As a pediatric rheumatologist, I often see children who have joint pain or swelling that's the result of vitamin D deficiency and inadequate nutrition.

Signs of vitamin D deficiency in children include:

- Severe "growing pains"
- Joint pain or swelling
- Poor stamina
- Decreased activity
- Scoliosis

- Other bone and joint deformities
- Recurring infections
- Frequent cavities and/or gum disease
- Tonsillitis
- Some forms of asthma

Q: People who keep all-year tans must be perfect examples of enough vitamin D, right? So if you're very tan, you're the epitome of health, or you just have very sun-damaged skin; and if you're very pale, you're D-deficient?

A: This is the paradox. The darker your skin and the faster you tan, the *more* sun you need to make enough vitamin D. Melanin is a natural sunscreen whose production is stimulated by sun (primarily UVA) exposure. Fair-skinned people are more efficient at making vitamin D than dark-skinned people. Someone with a dark complexion who isn't tanning or working out of doors is usually D-deficient.

Q: If we do *need* sun rays, why have dermatologists been scaring us for decades about too much sun—and telling people to cover up and slather on lots of sunscreen?

A: In an effort to make a public health message simple, we often throw the baby out with the bathwater. Remember when all fat was bad and the media touted no-fat diets? Remember when all carbs were bad? Now we know there are good fats and bad fats. Now we know that there are good carbohydrates and bad carbohydrates. As science progresses and as public knowledge increases, the message becomes more complex.

You do need the sun—there is no life on earth without it. But you're not choosing between no sun and *all the sun you want.* Regular intermittent exposure year round allows you to build up some melanin, which will buffer you from overexposure. Now-and-then sun exposure raises your vitamin D levels. Also, your skin type dictates how much sun you can tolerate. Avoid sunburns and think of clothing and sunscreen as tools that help to prevent sunburns and can reduce sun damage. The charts in chapter 5 will show you how to maximize sun exposure and vitamin D and minimize risk.

Q: Please explain the difference in the kinds of sun rays and what that means to our health. We need UVA or UVB or both or what?

A: The three spectrums of ultraviolet light are A, B, and C. All UVC is absorbed in the ozone. Small amounts of UVB penetrate the ozone, depending on its thickness, the angle of the sun, cloud cover, upper atmospheric changes, and solar activity. The variable that dominates the changes in UVB that pass through the ozone is the angle of the sun relative to you. The UVA spectrum penetrates the ozone year round.

- UVB—You need a modest amount daily or several times a week to make vitamin D.
- UVA—You can't avoid UVA if you go outside because this is the dominant UV light in our atmosphere.
- UVC—You get UVC only from artificial sources; it is not healthy.

Q: How important is it to eat organic?

A: This can be a very expensive step in the move toward a healthy lifestyle. Before focusing on organic foods, balance the acid-base in your diet and normalize your nutrient intake. You also can grow your own garden vegetables without pesticides or fertilizers or participate in community-supported agriculture (www.localharvest.org): you buy a share in a local organic farm before the growing season, then pick up your allotment of fresh produce weekly as you move through the harvests. Many organic farms also raise organic chickens, turkeys, and larger livestock. You can buy eggs from these farms and butcher your own meat (www.eatwild.com). More important than buying organic is to buy from local farmers.

The Right Vitamin D Tests

If you decide to get tested, work with your physician on your game plan. For the most exact dosing, you may want to have three blood tests; vitamin D_3, intact PTH (parathyroid hormone), and calcium.

The only way to know your vitamin D status definitively is to measure a blood level of 25-hydroxy-vitamin D_3. Your blood maintains activated vitamin D (also known as 1, 25-dihydroxyvitamin D_3) at a relatively constant level even when you're deficient in vitamin D. Activated D levels are a better measure of kidney function than vitamin D status.

Most lab tests adequately measure 25-hydroxy-vitamin D_3. However, physicians commonly use vitamin D_2, or ergocalciferol, to replace severe deficiencies. This form of D comes from plants, and most labs don't measure it accurately. This is important because underestimating the blood level of both forms of vitamin D may lead to overestimating what you need for D replacement; then concerns about toxicity may arise.

The DiaSorin method and HPLC (high-performance liquid chromatography) verified with tandem mass spectroscopy are the two methods that measure both forms of vitamin D. The DiaSorin method reports these as a single number, and the HPLC method reports D_2 and D_3 separately and as a total. These are the best methods of measurement that are widely available today. Both methods require quality controls to ensure accurate measures, and they should be periodically tested against each other relative to a standard.

Laboratory Corporation of America (LabCorp Inc.) is the largest commercial laboratory using primarily the Diasorin method of measurement. Mayo Clinic Laboratories and Quest Diagnostics are the two large labs that primarily use the HPLC dual mass spec method of measurement. Local hospital systems sometimes measure vitamin D in-house, or they send their tests to one of the large companies.

Assumptions about vitamin D status that are based on age, weight, occupation, supplementation level, and amount of sun exposure aren't as accurate as blood levels because the former can overestimate or underestimate a person's vitamin D status. Although adults fifty or older are at greatest risk, increased reports of rickets in the past decade show how vulnerable infants and children are. Some obese people are very physically active and spend a lot of time outdoors, which dilutes the risk of vitamin D deficiency inherent in being overweight. If you're unsure of your risk based on risk factors alone, measure your blood level.

The next blood test I recommend measures parathyroid hormone level (PTH). PTH comes from the parathyroid gland, which is different from the thyroid gland. PTH regulates calcium and phosphorus metabolism. When calcium or vitamin D levels fall or when phosphorus levels rise, PTH levels rise, too.

Rising phosphorus levels are typically associated with falling calcium levels. These two findings most commonly accompany kidney failure. If you are unsure about your kidney function, have that checked, too.

Phosphorus comes primarily from protein sources; that protein can come from your diet or your bones and muscles. High-protein diets without adequate produce theoretically can cause you to lose greater amounts of calcium in your urine, which may raise PTH levels; we see this almost exclusively in people with impaired kidney function. More commonly we see deficient dietary protein, which signals other hormones to pull phosphorus from bones and muscle, and this raises PTH levels.

A normal PTH level is between 10 and 65. But an ideal PTH level is between 10 and 40; the preferred level is below 40. With higher levels, your body will begin to sap calcium and phosphorus from the bone and put it into your bloodstream.

The three reasons you should measure your PTH and calcium are to identify

1. primary hyperparathyroidism;
2. other causes of high blood calcium levels; and
3. dietary imbalance and deficiencies.

Primary hyperparathyroidism comes from a tumor of the parathyroid gland that overproduces PTH. This often causes high calcium levels that will soar higher if you begin supplementing vitamin D and/or calcium. You need to correct this problem before you replace vitamin D or calcium. If you have a parathyroid tumor, you probably will be referred to a head and neck surgeon, who can remove this tumor.

One reason why it's important to identify other causes of high blood calcium levels is that sometimes bone pain related to cancer is accompanied by high calcium levels. Lung cancer, prostate cancer, breast cancer, and multiple myeloma all can cause bone pain and elevated calcium levels. Sarcoidosis—an immune-mediated disease—can cause elevated calcium levels, too.

The most common abnormalities that stimulate PTH production are calcium deficiency and insufficient dietary protein. Chronic dietary acidosis and vitamin D deficiency deplete calcium and magnesium stores. Protein malnutrition mobilizes phosphorus from bone and muscle. Parathyroid gland enlargement from these long-standing imbalances causes a persistently elevated PTH level that may take months to normalize despite replacement of vitamin D. Invariably these high PTH levels are accompanied by normal blood levels of calcium. The priorities remain the same. You need to normalize vitamin D levels; balance dietary acid-base; and replenish protein, magnesium, and calcium. The PTH level will eventually return to normal.

People with very low vitamin D levels often have normal PTH levels. They are either consuming lots of calcium, or they have significant magnesium deficiency. Magnesium is required to produce PTH, so in severe magnesium depletion, PTH levels won't rise in response to very low vitamin D levels. Furthermore, these individuals may be relatively vitamin D-resistant because magnesium is required for vitamin D to function properly. Magnesium replacement in vitamin D deficiency through diet or supplementation is critical and is as important as replenishing calcium stores.

Remember, if you have questions about your lab results, consult with the family physician or specialist (endocrinologist or rheumatologist) who's doing your evaluation. Let him or her know you're planning to take supplements.

Acid-Producing Levels of Different Foods

PREDICTED ACID-BASE FOR DIFFERENT FOOD GROUPS*	
Food Group	Potential Renal Acid Load
Beverages (avg.)	0.00
Milk	1.00
Mineral water	−1.60
Soft drink	0.40
Tea	−0.30
Beer, pale	0.90
Beer, stout	−0.10
Wine, red	−2.40
Wine, white	−1.20
Fish (avg.)	7.90
Meat (avg.)	9.50
Nuts (avg.)	7.00
Peanuts	8.30
Walnuts	6.80
Hazelnuts	−2.80

Food Group	Potential Renal Acid Load
Grains (avg.)	5.50
Bread	4.00
Flour	7.00
Pasta	6.70
Corn flakes	6.00
Oat flakes	10.70
Dairy (cheese avg.)	23.40
Cheddar, low-fat	26.40
Cottage cheese	8.70
Hard cheese (avg.)	19.20
Parmesan	34.20
Processed cheese	28.70
Other Dairy	
Whey	−1.60
Yogurt with fruit	1.20
Fruits and Fruit Juice (avg.)	−3.10
Apples	−2.20
Bananas	−5.50
Cherries	−3.60
Lemon juice	−2.50
Orange juice	−2.90
Peaches	−2.40
Raisins	−21.00
Vegetables (avg.)	−2.80
Asparagus	−0.40
Broccoli	−1.20
Carrots	−4.90
Cucumbers	−0.80
Lettuce	−2.50
Mushrooms	−1.40
Onions	−1.50
Potatoes	−4.00
Spinach	−14.00
Tomatoes	−3.10
Zucchini	−4.60

*Serving size is 100 grams, or about 3.5 ounces by weight.
Adapted from Remer T, Manz F. Potential renal acid load of foods and its influence on urine pH. *J Am Diet Assoc.* 1995 Jul; 95(7): 791–7.

Online Resources

Food

www.localharvest.org—An invaluable resource for local meats, vegetables, fruits, and more. This website will connect you to the farmers in your area.

www.eatwild.com—The focus of this site is to help you locate farms nationwide that provide grass-fed or free-range livestock.

www.tastesmilerepeat.com—Chef Kelly, the creator of this book's fifteen new recipes and the two-week menu.

Vitamin D and Other Supplements

www.carlsonlabs.com—Specialists in fat-soluble vitamins and fish oil products.

www.ddrops.ca—The most accurate liquid vitamin D delivery system.

www.evitamins.com—Family-owned online vitamin retailer located in Michigan.

www.jarrowformulas.com—Founder-owned and operated since 1977. Formulates and manufactures its own line of supplements and distributes worldwide.

www.nowfoods.com—Family-owned supplement manufacturer since 1968, with A-rated good manufacturing practices from the Natural Products Association, distributed locally and online.

www.swansonvitamins.com—Family-owned online catalog vitamin company established in 1969, with some of the best prices on its own brands as well as others.

Vitamin D Testing

www.labcorp.com

www.questdiagnostics.com

www.mayomedicallaboratories.com

www.zrtlab.com (self-testing)

Paleolithic Recipes

www.thevitamindcure.com

www.thepaleodiet.com

Ultraviolet Lights

www.sperti.com—Makes UVB lamps specifically for the purpose of raising your vitamin D level.

Weather Information

www.cpc.ncep.noaa.gov/products/stratosphere/uv_index/uv_annual .shtml—United States annual UV-index maps by city.

http://www.epa.gov/sunwise/uvicalc.html—Explains how UV index is calculated and provides a tool to calculate UV index at your zip code.

http://apps.usa.gov/uvindex/—Download an app for your mobile device that determines your local UV index.

www.wunderground.com—Local weather from local folks—includes UV index estimate for that day.

References

Abate N, Chandalia M, Cabo-Chan AV Jr., Moe OW, Sakhaee K. The metabolic syndrome and uric acid nephrolithiasis: novel features of renal manifestation of insulin resistance. *Kidney Int.* 2004 Feb;65(2):386–92.

Abbas S, Linseisen J, Slanger T, et al. Serum 25-hydroxyvitamin D and risk of post-menopausal breast cancer—results of a large case-control study. *Carcinogenesis.* 2008;29:93–9.

Abbott RD, Ando F, Masaki KH, Tung KH, Rodriguez BL, Petrovitch H, Yano K, Curb JD. Dietary magnesium intake and the future risk of coronary heart disease (the Honolulu Heart Program). *Am J Cardiol.* 2003 Sep 15;92(6): 665–9.

Adams J, Hewison M. Unexpected actions of vitamin D: new perspectives on the regulation of innate and adaptive immunity. *Nat Clin Pract Endocrinol Metab.* 2008;4(2):80–90.

Adler GK, Geenen R. Hypothalamic-pituitary-adrenal and autonomic nervous system functioning in fibromyalgia. *Rheum Dis Clin North Am.* 2005 Feb;31 (1):187–202.

Adorini L, Penna J. Control of autoimmune diseases by the vitamin D endocrine system. *Nature Clin Pract Rheum.* 2008;4(8):404–12.

Adorini L, Penna G, Giarratana N, Uskokovic M. Tolerogenic dendritic cells induced by vitamin D receptor ligands enhance regulatory T-cells inhibiting allograft rejection and autoimmune diseases. *J Cell Biochem.* 2003 Feb 1;88(2):227–33.

Agus ZS. Hypomagnesemia. *J Am Soc Nephrol.* 1999 Jul;10(7):1616–22.

Aihara K, Azuma H, Akaike M, Ikeda Y, Yamashita M, Sudo T, Hayashi H, Yamada Y, Endoh F, Fujimura M, Yoshida T, Yamaguchi H, Hashizume S, Kato M, Yoshimura K, Yamamoto Y, Kato S, Matsumoto T. Disruption of nuclear vitamin D receptor gene causes enhanced thrombogenicity in mice. *J Biol Chem.* 2004 Aug 20;279(34):35798–802. Epub 2004 Jun 17.

Al Faraj S, Al Mutairi K. Vitamin D deficiency and chronic low back pain in Saudi Arabia. *Spine.* 2003 Jan 15;28(2):177–9.

Alberts DS, Martinez ME, Roe DJ, Guillen-Rodriguez JM, Marshall JR, van Leeuwen JB, Reid ME, et al. Lack of effect of a high-fiber cereal supplement on the recurrence of colorectal adenomas. Phoenix Colon Cancer Prevention Physicians' Network. *N Engl J Med.* 2000 Apr 20;342(16):1156–62.

Alexy U, Remer T, Manz F, Neu CM, Schoenau E. Long-term protein intake and dietary potential renal acid load are associated with bone modeling and remodeling at the proximal radius in healthy children. *Am J Clin Nutr.* 2005 Nov;82(5):1107–14.

Andjelkovic Z, Vojinovic J, Pejnovic N, Popovic M, Dujic A, Mitrovic D, Pavlica L, Stefanovic D. Disease modifying and immunomodulatory effects of high dose 1 alpha (OH) D3 in rheumatoid arthritis patients. *Clin Exp Rheumatol.* 1999 Jul–Aug;17(4):453–6.

Appel LJ, Moore TJ, Obarzanek E, Vollmer WM, Svetkey LP, Sacks FM, et al. A clinical trial of the effects of dietary patterns on blood pressure. DASH Collaborative Research Group. *N Engl J Med.* 1997 Apr 17;336(16):1117–24.

Aranda A, Pascual A. Nuclear hormone receptors and gene expression. *Physiol Rev.* 2001 Jul;81(3):1269–304.

Ard JD, Grambow SC, Liu D, Slentz CA, Kraus WE, Svetkey LP; PREMIER study. The effect of the PREMIER interventions on insulin sensitivity. *Diabetes Care.* 2004 Feb;27(2):340–7.

Arlt W, Fremerey C, Callies F, Reincke M, Schneider P, Timmermann W, Allolio B. Well-being, mood, and calcium homeostasis in patients with hypoparathyroidism receiving standard treatment with calcium and vitamin D. *Eur J Endocrinol.* 2002 Feb;146(2):215–22.

Armitage EL, Aldhous MC, Anderson N, Drummond HE, Riemersma RA, Ghosh S, Satsangi J. Incidence of juvenile-onset Crohn's disease in Scotland: association with northern latitude and affluence. *Gastroenterology.* 2004 Oct;127(4):1051–7.

Armitage JA, Taylor PD, Poston L. Experimental models of developmental programming: consequences of exposure to an energy-rich diet during development. *J Physiol.* 2005 May 15;565(Pt 1):3–8.

Arterburn LM, Hall EB, Oken H. Distribution, interconversion, and dose response of n-3 fatty acids in humans. *Am J Clin Nutr.* 2006 Jun;83(6 Suppl):1467S–1476S.

Arunabh S, Pollack S, Yeh J, Aloia JF. Body fat content and 25-hydroxyvitamin D levels in healthy women. *J Clin Endocrinol Metab.* 2003 Jan;88(1):157–61.

Azadbakht L, Mirmiran P, Esmaillzadeh A, Azizi T, Azizi F. Beneficial effects of a Dietary Approaches to Stop Hypertension eating plan on features of the metabolic syndrome. *Diabetes Care.* 2005 Dec;28(12):2823–31.

Baba N, Samson S, Bouurdet-Sicard R, Rubio M, Sarfati M. Commensal bacteria trigger a full dendritic cell maturation program that promotes the expansion of non-Tr1 suppressor T cells (Treg). *J Leuk Biol.* 2008;84(2):468–76.

Backstrom MC, Maki R, Kuusela AL, Sievanen H, Koivisto AM, Ikonen RS, Kouri T, Maki M. Randomised controlled trial of vitamin D supplementation on bone density and biochemical indices in preterm infants. *Arch Dis Child Fetal Neonatal Ed.* 1999 May;80(3):F161–6.

Balato A, Unutmaz D, Gaspari A. Natural killer T cells: an unconventional T-cell subset with diverse effector and regulatory functions. *J Invest Derm.* 2009;129:1628–42.

Banchereau J, Pascual V, Palucka AK. Autoimmunity through cytokine-induced dendritic cell activation. *Immunity.* 2004 May;20(5):539–50.

Barger-Lux MJ, Davies KM, Heaney RP. Calcium supplementation does not augment bone gain in young women consuming diets moderately low in calcium. *J Nutr.* 2005 Oct;135(10):2362–6.

Barreto AM, Schwartz GG, Woodruff R, Cramer SD. 25-Hydroxyvitamin D₃, the pro-hormone of 1,25-dihydroxyvitamin D₃, inhibits the proliferation of primary prostatic epithelial cells. *Cancer Epidemiol Biomarkers Prev.* 2000 Mar;9(3):265–70.

Becker A, Eyles DW, McGrath JJ, Grecksch G. Transient prenatal vitamin D deficiency is associated with subtle alterations in learning and memory functions in adult rats. *Behav Brain Res.* 2005 Jun 20;161(2):306–12.

Belderbos ME, Houben ML, Wilbrink B, Lentjes E, Bloemen EM, Kimpen JL, Rovers M, Bont L. Cord blood vitamin D deficiency is associated with respiratory syncytial virus bronchiolitis. *Pediatrics.* 2011 May 9. Jun;127(6):e1513–1520.

Bengtsson AK, Ryan EJ, Giordano D, Magaletti DM, Clark EA. 17 beta-estradiol (E2) modulates cytokine and chemokine expression in human monocyte-derived dendritic cells. *Blood.* 2004 Sep 1;104(5):1404–10.

Bennett RM, Lehr JR, McCarty DJ. Factors affecting the solubility of calcium pyrophosphate dihydrate crystals. *J Clin Invest.* 1975 Dec;56(6):1571–9.

Bergink AP, Uitterlinden AG, Van Leeuwen JP, Buurman CJ, Hofman A, Verhaar JA, Pols HA. Vitamin D status, bone mineral density, and the development of radiographic osteoarthritis of the knee: the Rotterdam Study. *J Clin Rheumatol.* 2009 Aug;15(5):230–7.

Bertone-Johnson ER. Vitamin D and the occurrence of depression: causal association or circumstantial evidence? *Nutr Rev.* 2009 Aug;67(8):481–92.

Bertone-Johnson ER, Chen WY, Holick MF, Hollis BW, Colditz GA, Willett WC, Hankinson SE. Plasma 25-hydroxyvitamin D and 1,25-dihydroxyvitamin D and risk of breast cancer. *Cancer Epidemiol Biomarkers Prev.* 2005 Aug;14(8):1991–7.

Berwick M, Armstrong BK, Ben-Porat L, Fine J, Kricker A, Eberle C, Barnhill R. Sun exposure and mortality from melanoma. *J Natl Cancer Inst.* 2005 Feb 2;97(3):195–9.

Bhargava SK, Sachdev HS, Fall CH, Osmond C, Lakshmy R, Barker DJ, Biswas SK, Ramji S, Prabhakaran D, Reddy KS. Relation of serial changes in childhood body-mass index to impaired glucose tolerance in young adulthood. *N Engl J Med.* 2004 Feb 26;350(9):865–75.

Bichara M, Mercier O, Borensztein P, Paillard M. Acute metabolic acidosis enhances circulating parathyroid hormone, which contributes to the renal response against acidosis in the rat. *J Clin Invest.* 1990 Aug;86(2):430–43.

Bigal ME, Bordini CA, Tepper SJ, Speciali JG. Intravenous magnesium sulphate in the acute treatment of migraine without aura and migraine with aura. A randomized, double-blind, placebo-controlled study. *Cephalalgia.* 2002 Jun;22(5):345–53.

Bischoff-Ferrari HA, Dawson-Hughes B, Baron JA, Burckhardt P, Li R, Spiegelman D, et al. Calcium intake and hip fracture risk in men and women: a meta-analysis of prospective cohort studies and randomized controlled trials. *Am J Clin Nutr.* 2007;86:1780–90.

Bischoff-Ferrari HA, Dawson-Hughes B, Staehelin HB, Orav JE, Stuck AE, Theiler R, Wong JB, Egli A, Kiel DP, Henschkowski J. Fall prevention with supplemental and active forms of vitamin D: a meta-analysis of randomized controlled trials. *BMJ.* 2009 Oct 1;339:3692–703.

Bischoff-Ferrari HA, Dawson-Hughes B, Willett WC, Staehelin HB, Bazemore MG, Zee RY, Wong JB. Effect of vitamin D on falls: a meta-analysis. *JAMA.* 2004 Apr 28;291(16):1999–2006.

Bischoff-Ferrari HA, Dietrich T, Orav EJ, Dawson-Hughes B. Positive association between 25-hydroxyvitamin D levels and bone mineral density: a population-based study of younger and older adults. *Am J Med.* 2004 May 1;116(9):634–9.

Bischoff-Ferrari HA, Dietrich T, Orav EJ, Hu FB, Zhang Y, Karlson EW, Dawson-Hughes B. Higher 25-hydroxyvitamin D concentrations are associated with better lower-extremity function in both active and inactive persons aged > or =60 y. *Am J Clin Nutr.* 2004 Sep;80(3):752–8.

Bischoff-Ferrari HA, Giovannucci E, Willett WC, Dietrich T, Dawson-Hughes B. Estimation of optimal serum concentrations of 25-hydroxyvitamin D for multiple health outcomes. *Am J Clin Nutr.* 2006 Jul;84(1):18–28.

Bischoff-Ferrari HA, Willett WC, Wong JB, Giovannucci E, Dietrich T, Dawson-Hughes B. Fracture prevention with vitamin D supplementation: a meta-analysis of randomized controlled trials. *JAMA.* 2005 May 11;293(18):2257–64.

Black PN, Scragg R. Relationship between serum 25-hydroxyvitamin D and pulmonary function in the third national health and nutrition examination survey. *Chest.* 2005 Dec;128(6):3792–8.

Blair SN, LaMonte MJ, Nichaman MZ. The evolution of physical activity recommendations: how much is enough? *Am J Clin Nutr.* 2004 May;79(5): 913S–920S.

Blanco P, Palucka AK, Gill M, Pascual V, Banchereau J. Induction of dendritic cell differentiation by IFN-alpha in systemic lupus erythematosus. *Science.* 2001 Nov 16;294(5546):1540–3.

Blanco P, Palucka AK, Pascual V, Banchereau J. Dendritic cells and cytokines in human inflammatory and autoimmune diseases. *Cytokines Growth Factor Rev.* 2008 February;19(1):41–52.

Blois S, Kammerrer U, Soto C, et al. Dendritic cells: key to fetal tolerance? *Biol Reprod.* 2007;77:590–8.

Bloomfield FH, Oliver MH, Hawkins P, Holloway AC, Campbell M, Gluckman PD, Harding JE, Challis JR. Periconceptional undernutrition in sheep accelerates maturation of the fetal hypothalamic-pituitary-adrenal axis in late gestation. *Endocrinology.* 2004 Sep;145(9):4278–85.

Blow FC, Zeber JE, McCarthy JF, Valenstein M, Gillon L, Bingham CR. Ethnicity and diagnostic patterns in veterans with psychoses. *Soc Psychiatry Psychiatr Epidemiol.* 2004 Oct;39(10):841–51.

Bodnar LM, Catov JM, Simhan HN, Holick MF, Powers RW, Roberts JM. Maternal vitamin D deficiency increases the risk of preeclampsia. *J Clin Endocrinol Metab.* 2007 Sep;92(9):3517–22.

Bodnar LM, Simhan HN, Powers RW, Frank MP Cooperstein E, Roberts JM. High prevalence of vitamin D deficiency in black and white pregnant women residing in the northern United States and their neonates. *J Nutr.* 2007 Feb;137(2):447–52.

Bolland MJ, Avenell A, Baron JA, Grey A, MacLennan GS, Gamble GD, Reid IR. Effect of calcium supplements on risk of myocardial infarction and cardiovascular events: meta-analysis. *BMJ.* 2010 Jul 29;341:c3691.

Borissova AM, Tankova T, Kirilov G, Dakovska L, Kovacheva R. The effect of vitamin D_3 on insulin secretion and peripheral insulin sensitivity in type 2 diabetic patients. *Int J Clin Pract.* 2003 May;57(4):258–61.

Boscoe FP, Schymura MJ. Solar ultraviolet-B exposure and cancer incidence and mortality in the United States, 1993–2002. *BMC Cancer.* 2006 Nov 10;6:264.

Boska MD, Welch KM, Barker PB, Nelson JA, Schultz L. Contrasts in cortical magnesium, phospholipids, and energy metabolism between migraine syndromes. *Neurology.* 2002 Apr 23;58(8):1227–33.

Bourlioux P, Koletzko B, Guarner F, Braesco V. The intestine and its microflora are partners for the protection of the host: report on the Danone Symposium "The Intelligent Intestine," held in Paris, June 14, 2002. *Am J Clin Nutr.* 2003 Oct;78(4):675–83.

Brewer LD, Thibault V, Chen KC, Langub MC, Landfield PW, Porter NM. Vitamin D hormone confers neuroprotection in parallel with downregulation of L-type calcium channel expression in hippocampal neurons. *J Neurosci.* 2001 Jan 1;21(1):98–108.

Brooke OG, Brown IR, Bone CD, Carter ND, Cleeve HJ, Maxwell JD, Robinson VP, Winder SM. Vitamin D supplements in pregnant Asian women: effects on calcium status and fetal growth. *Br Med J.* 1980 Mar 15;280(6216): 751–4.

Brooke OG, Butters F, Wood C. Intrauterine vitamin D nutrition and postnatal growth in Asian infants. *Br Med J (Clin Res Ed).* 1981 Oct 17;283(6298): 1024.

Brot C, Jorgensen NR, Sorensen OH. The influence of smoking on vitamin D status and calcium metabolism. *Eur J Clin Nutr.* 1999 Dec;53(12): 920–6.

Buell JS, Dawson-Hughes B, Scott TM, Weiner DE, Dallal GE, Qui WQ, Bergethon P, Rosenberg IH, Folstein MF, Patz S, Bhadelia RA, Tucker KL. 25-Hydroxyvitamin D, dementia, and cerebrovascular pathology in elders receiving home services. *Neurology.* 2010 Jan 5;74(1):18–26.

Buell JS, Dawson-Hughes B. Vitamin D and neurocognitive dysfunction: preventing "D"ecline? *Mol Aspects Med.* 2008 Dec;29(6):415–22.

Buell JS, Scott TM, Dawson-Hughes B, Dallal GE, Rosenberg IH, Folstein MF, Tucker KL. Vitamin D is associated with cognitive function in elders receiving home health services. *J Gerontol A Biol Sci Med Sci.* 2009 Aug;64(8):888–95.

Burton JM, Kimball S, Vieth R, Bar-Or A, Dosch HM, Cheung R, Gagne D, D'Souza C, Ursell M, O'Connor P. A phase I/II dose-escalation trial of vitamin D3 and calcium in multiple sclerosis. *Neurology.* 2010 Jun 8;74(23):1852–9.

Bushinsky DA. Acid-base imbalance and the skeleton. *Eur J Nutr.* 2001 Oct;40(5):238–44.

Cade C, Norman AW. Vitamin D_3 improves impaired glucose tolerance and insulin secretion in the vitamin D–deficient rat in vivo. *Endocrinology.* 1986 Jul;119(1):84–90.

Calder PC. N-3 polyunsaturated fatty acids, inflammation, and inflammatory diseases. *Am J Clin Nutr.* 2006 Jun;83(6 Suppl):1505S–1519S.

Camargo CA Jr, Rifas-Shiman SL, Litonjua AA, Rich-Edwards JW, Weiss ST, Gold DR, Kleinman K, Gillman MW. Maternal intake of vitamin D during pregnancy and risk of recurrent wheeze in children at 3 y of age. *Am J Clin Nutr.* 2007 Mar;85(3):788–95.

Campbell MJ, Gombart AF, Kwok SH, Park S, Koeffler HP. The anti-proliferative effects of 1alpha,25(OH)2D3 on breast and prostate cancer cells are associated with induction of BRCA1 gene expression. *Oncogene.* 2000;19(44):5091–7.

Cannell JJ, Vieth R, Umhau JC, Holick MF, Grant WB, Madronich S, Garland CF, Giovannucci E. Epidemic influenza and vitamin D. *Epidemiol Infect.* 2006 Dec;134(6):1129–40. Epub 2006 Sep 7.

Cantorna MT, Hayes CE, DeLuca HF. 1,25-Dihydroxycholecalciferol inhibits the progression of arthritis in murine models of human arthritis. *J Nutr.* 1998 Jan;128(1):68–72.

———. 1,25-Dihydroxyvitamin D_3 reversibly blocks the progression of relapsing encephalomyelitis, a model of multiple sclerosis. *Proc Natl Acad Sci USA.* 1996 Jul 23;93(15):7861–4.

Cantorna MT, Mahon BD. Mounting evidence for vitamin D as an environmental factor affecting autoimmune disease prevalence. *Exp Biol Med (Maywood).* 2004 Dec;229(11):1136–42.

Cantorna MT, Munsick C, Bemiss C, Mahon BD. 1,25-dihydroxycholecalciferol prevents and ameliorates symptoms of experimental murine inflammatory bowel disease. *J Nutr.* 2000 Nov;130(11):2648–52.

Cantorna MT, Zhu Y, Froicu M, Wittke A. Vitamin D status, 1,25-dihydroxyvitamin D_3, and the immune system. *Am J Clin Nutr.* 2004 Dec; 80(6 Suppl):1717S–20S.

Cardus A, Parisi E, Gallego C, Aldea M, Fernandez E, Valdivielso JM. 1,25-dihydroxyvitamin D3 stimulates vascular smooth muscle cell proliferation through a VEGF mediated pathway. *Kidney Int.* 2006;69:1377–84.

Carpentier YA, Portois L, Malaisse WJ. N-3 fatty acids and the metabolic syndrome. *Am J Clin Nutr.* 2006 Jun;83(6 Suppl):1499S–1504S.

Chacko SA, Song Y, Manson JE, Van Horn L, Eaton C, Martin LW, McTiernan A, Curb JD, Wylie-Rosett J, Phillips LS, Plodkowski RA, Liu S. Serum 25-hydroxyvitamin D concentrations in relation to cardiometabolic risk factors and metabolic syndrome in postmenopausal women. *Am J Clin Nutr.* 2011 Jul;94(1):209–17.

Chaganti RK, Parimi N, Cawthon P, Dam TL, Nevitt MC, Lane NE. Association of 25-hydroxyvitamin D with prevalent osteoarthritis of the hip in elderly men: the osteoporotic fractures in men study. *Arthritis Rheum.* 2010 Feb;62(2):511–4.

Chan She Ping-Delfos W, Soares M. Diet induced thermogenesis, fat oxidation and food intake following sequential meals: influence of calcium and vitamin D. *Clin Nutr.* 2011 Jan 26.

Chapuy MC, Arlot ME, Duboeuf F, Brun J, Crouzet B, Arnaud S, Delmas PD, Meunier PJ. Vitamin D_3 and calcium to prevent hip fractures in the elderly women. *N Engl J Med.* 1992 Dec 3;327(23):1637–42.

Chapuy MC, Pamphile R, Paris E, Kempf C, Schlichting M, Arnaud S, Garnero P, Meunier PJ. Combined calcium and vitamin D_3 supplementation in elderly women: confirmation of reversal of secondary hyperparathyroidism and hip fracture risk: the Decalyos II study. *Osteoporos Int.* 2002 Mar;13(3): 257–64.

Chen S, Sims GP, Chen XX, Gu YY, Chen S, Lipsky PE. Modulatory effects of 1,25-dihydroxyvitamin D3 on human B cell differentiation. *J Immunol.* 2007 Aug 1;179(3):1634–47.

Cheng S, Massaro JM, Fox CS, Larson MG, Keyes MJ, McCabe EL, Robins SJ, O'Donnell CJ, Hoffmann U, Jacques PF, Booth SL, Vasan RS, Wolf M, Wang TJ. Adiposity, cardiometabolic risk, and vitamin D status: the Framingham Heart Study. *Diabetes.* 2010;59:242–8.

Cheng S, Tylavsky F, Kroger H, Karkkainen M, Lyytikainen A, Koistinen A, Mahonen, et al. Association of low 25-hydroxyvitamin D concentrations with elevated parathyroid hormone concentrations and low cortical bone density in early pubertal and prepubertal Finnish girls. *Am J Clin Nutr.* 2003 Sep;78 (3):485–92.

Chiu KC, Chu A, Go VL, Saad MF. Hypovitaminosis D is associated with insulin resistance and beta cell dysfunction. *Am J Clin Nutr.* 2004 May;79 (5):820–5.

Choi HK, Atkinson K, Karlson EW, Willett W, Curhan G. Purine-rich foods, dairy and protein intake, and the risk of gout in men. *N Engl J Med.* 2004 Mar 11;350(11):1093–103.

Christensen R, Astrup A, Bliddal H. Weight loss: the treatment of choice for knee osteoarthritis? A randomized trial. *Osteoarthritis Cartilage.* 2005 Jan;13(1):20–7.

Colston K, Colston MJ, Feldman D. 1,25-dihydroxyvitamin D_3 and malignant melanoma: the presence of receptors and inhibition of cell growth in culture. *Endocrinology.* 1981 Mar;108(3):1083–6.

Conigrave AD, Mun HC, Delbridge L, Quinn SJ, Wilkinson M, Brown EM. L-amino acids regulate parathyroid hormone secretion. *J Biol Chem.* 2004 Sep 10;279(37):38151–9. Epub 2004 Jul 2.

Cordain L, Eaton SB, Miller JB, Mann N, Hill K. The paradoxical nature of hunter-gatherer diets: meat-based, yet non-atherogenic. *Eur J Clin Nutr.* 2002 Mar;56 Suppl 1:S42–52.

Cordain L, Eaton SB, Sebastian A, Mann N, Lindeberg S, Watkins BA, O'Keefe JH, Brand-Miller J. Origins and evolution of the Western diet: health implications for the 21st century. *Am J Clin Nutr.* 2005 Feb;81(2):341–54.

Cox IM, Campbell MJ, Dowson D. Red blood cell magnesium and chronic fatigue syndrome. *Lancet.* 1991 Mar 30;337(8744):757–60.

Crosby V, Wilcock A, Corcoran R. The safety and efficacy of a single dose (500 mg or 1 g) of intravenous magnesium sulfate in neuropathic pain poorly responsive to strong opioid analgesics in patients with cancer. *J Pain Symptom Manage.* 2000 Jan;19(1):35–9.

Dawson-Hughes B, Harris SS, Krall EA, Dallal GE. Effect of calcium and vitamin D supplementation on bone density in men and women 65 years of age or older. *N Engl J Med.* 1997 Sep 4;337(10):670–6.

Dawson-Hughes B, Harris SS, Rasmussen H, Song L, Dallal GE. Effect of dietary protein supplements on calcium excretion in healthy older men and women. *J Clin Endocrinol Metab.* 2004 Mar;89(3):1169–73.

Daynes RA, Enioutina EY, Butler S, Mu HH, McGee ZA, Araneo BA. Induction of common mucosal immunity by hormonally immunomodulated peripheral immunization. *Infect Immun.* 1996 Apr;64(4):1100–9.

de Lorgeril M, Salen P, Martin JL, Mamelle N, Monjaud I, Touboul P, Delaye J. Effect of a Mediterranean type of diet on the rate of cardiovascular complications in patients with coronary artery disease: insights into the cardioprotective effect of certain nutrients. *J Am Coll Cardiol.* 1996 Nov 1;28(5):1103–8.

de Lorgeril M, Salen P, Martin JL, Monjaud I, Boucher P, Mamelle N. Mediterranean dietary pattern in a randomized trial: prolonged survival and possible reduced cancer rate. *Arch Intern Med.* 1998 Jun 8;158(11):1181–7.

de Lorgeril M, Salen P, Martin JL, Monjaud I, Delaye J, Mamelle N. Mediterranean diet, traditional risk factors, and the rate of cardiovascular complications after myocardial infarction: final report of the Lyon Diet Heart Study. *Circulation.* 1999 Feb 16;99(6):779–85.

DeLucia MC, Mitnick ME, Carpenter TO. Nutritional rickets with normal circulating 25-hydroxyvitamin D: a call for reexamining the role of dietary calcium intake in North American infants. *J Clin Endocrinol Metab.* 2003 Aug;88(8):3539–45.

Derex L, Trouillas P. Reversible parkinsonism, hypophosphoremia, and hypocalcemia under vitamin D therapy. *Mov Disord.* 1997 Jul;12(4):612–3.

Deroisy R, Collette J, Albert A, Jupsin I, Reginster JY. Administration of a supplement containing both calcium and vitamin D is more effective than calcium alone to reduce secondary hyperparathyroidism in postmenopausal women with low 25(OH) vitamin D circulating levels. *Aging Clin Exp Res.* 2002 Feb;14(1):13–7.

Devine A, Wilson SG, Dick IM, Prince RL. Effects of vitamin D metabolites on intestinal calcium absorption and bone turnover in elderly women. *Am J Clin Nutr.* 2002 Feb;75(2):283–8.

de Vogel J, Jonker-Termont DS, van Lieshout EM, Katan MB, van der Meer R. Green vegetables, red meat, and colon cancer: chlorophyll prevents the cytotoxic and hyperproliferative effects of haem in rat colon. *Carcinogenesis.* 2005 Feb;26(2):387–93.

Dietrich T, Joshipura KJ, Dawson-Hughes B, Bischoff-Ferrari HA. Association between serum concentrations of 25-hydroxyvitamin D_3 and periodontal disease in the US population. *Am J Clin Nutr.* 2004 Jul;80(1):108–13.

Dimai HP, Porta S, Wirnsberger G, Lindschinger M, Pamperl I, Dobnig H, Wilders-Truschnig M, Lau KH. Daily oral magnesium supplementation suppresses bone turnover in young adult males. *J Clin Endocrinol Metab.* 1998 Aug;83(8):2742–8.

Ding C, Cicuttini F, Parameswaran V, Burgess J, Quinn S, Jones G. Serum levels of vitamin D, sunlight exposure, and knee cartilage loss in older adults: the Tasmanian older adult cohort study. *Arthritis Rheum.* 2009 May;60(5):1381–9.

Dlugos DJ, Perrotta PL, Horn WG. Effects of the submarine environment on renal-stone risk factors and vitamin D metabolism. *Undersea Hyperb Med.* 1995 Jun;22(2):145–52.

Dobnig H, Pilz S, Scharnagl H, Renner W, Seelhorst U, Wellnitz B, Kinkeldei J, Boehm BO, Weihrauch G, Maerz W. Independent association of low serum 25-hydroxyvitamin D and 1,25-dihydroxyvitamin D levels with all-cause and cardiovascular mortality. *Arch Intern Med.* 2008;168:1340–9.

Eaton SB, Eaton SB III. Paleolithic vs. modern diets—selected pathophysiological implications. *Eur J Nutr.* 2000 Apr;39(2):67–70.

Eaton SB, Eaton SB III, Sinclair AJ, Cordain L, Mann NJ. Dietary intake of long-chain polyunsaturated fatty acids during the paleolithic period. *World Rev Nutr Diet.* 1998;83:12–23.

Eaton SB, Konner M. Paleolithic nutrition: a consideration of its nature and current implications. *N Engl J Med.* 1985 Jan 31;312(5):283–9.

Eide MJ, Weinstock MA. Association of UV index, latitude, and melanoma incidence in nonwhite populations—U.S. Surveillance, Epidemiology, and End Results (SEER) Program, 1992 to 2001. *Arch Dermatol.* 2005 Apr;141(4):477–81.

Elango R, Humayun MA, Ball RO, Pencharz PB. Evidence that protein requirements have been significantly underestimated. *Curr Opin Clin Nutr Metab Care.* 2010 Jan;13(1):52–7.

Elian M, Nightingale S, Dean G. Multiple sclerosis among United Kingdom–born children of immigrants from the Indian subcontinent, Africa, and the West Indies. *J Neurol Neurosurg Psychiatry.* 1990 Oct;53(10):906–11.

Endo I, Inoue D, Mitsui T, Umaki Y, Akaike M, Yoshizawa T, Kato S, Matsumoto T. Deletion of vitamin D receptor gene in mice results in abnormal skeletal muscle development with deregulated expression of myoregulatory transcription factors. *Endocrinology.* 2003 Dec;144(12):5138–44.

Enioutina EY, Visic D, McGee ZA, Daynes RA. The induction of systemic and mucosal immune responses following the subcutaneous immunization of mature adult mice: characterization of the antibodies in mucosal secretions of animals immunized with antigen formulations containing a vitamin D_3 adjuvant. *Vaccine.* 1999 Aug 6;17(23–24):3050–64.

Eriksson JG, Forsen T, Tuomilehto J, Osmond C, Barker DJ. Early growth and coronary heart disease in later life: longitudinal study. *BMJ.* 2001 Apr 21; 322(7292):949–53.

Eriksson JG, Osmond C, Kajantie E, Forsen TJ, Barker DJ. Patterns of growth among children who later develop type 2 diabetes or its risk factors. *Diabetologia.* 2006 Dec;49(12):2853–8. Epub 2006 Oct 3.

Esposito K, Marfella R, Ciotola M, Di Palo C, Giugliano F, Giugliano G, D'Armiento M, D'Andrea F, Giugliano D. Effect of a Mediterranean-style diet on endothelial dysfunction and markers of vascular inflammation in the metabolic syndrome: a randomized trial. *JAMA.* 2004 Sep 2;292(12): 1440–6.

Evans K, Nguyen L, Chan J. Effects of 25 hydroxyvitamin D3 and 1, 25 dihydroxy-vitamin D3 on cytokine production by human decidual cells. *Biology Reprod.* 2006; 75:816–22.

Eyles DW, Feron F, Cui X, Kesby JP, Harms LH, Ko P, McGrath JJ, Burne TH. Developmental vitamin D deficiency causes abnormal brain development. *Psychoneuroendocrinology.* 2009 Dec;34 Suppl 1:S247–S257.

Fang F, Kasperzyk JL, Shui I, Hendrickson W, Hollis BW, Fall K, Ma J, Gaziano JM, Stampfer MJ, Mucci LA, Giovannucci E. Prediagnostic plasma vitamin D metabolites and mortality among patients with prostate cancer. *PLoS One.* 2011 Apr 6;6(4):e18625.

Fernandes de Abreu DA, Eyles D, Féron F. Vitamin D, a neuro-immunomodulator: implications for neurodegenerative and autoimmune diseases. *Psychoneuroendocrinology.* 2009 Dec;34 Suppl 1:S265–S277.

Finch PJ, Ang L, Colston KW, Nisbet J, Maxwell JD. Blunted seasonal variation in serum 25-hydroxyvitamin D and increased risk of osteomalacia in vegetarian London Asians. *Eur J Clin Nutr.* 1992 Jul;46(7):509–15.

Forbes K, Westwood M. Maternal growth factor regulation in human placental development and fetal growth. *J Endocrinol.* 2010;207:1–16.

Ford ES, Ajani UA, McGuire LC, Liu S. Concentrations of serum vitamin D and the metabolic syndrome among U.S. adults. *Diabetes Care.* 2005 May;28(5): 1228–30.

Ford ES, Mokdad AH. Dietary magnesium intake in a national sample of U.S. adults. *J Nutr.* 2003 Sep;133(9):2879–82.

Forman JP, Giovannucci E, Holmes MD, Bischoff-Ferrari HA, Tworoger SS, Willett WC, Curhan GC. Plasma 25-hydroxyvitamin D levels and risk of incident hypertension. *Hypertension.* 2007;49:1063–9.

Fowden A, Forhead A. Endocrine regulation of feto-placental growth. *Hormone Res.* 2009;72:257–65.

Fox CH, Mahoney MC, Ramsoomair D, Carter CA. Magnesium deficiency in African-Americans: does it contribute to increased cardiovascular risk factors? *J Natl Med Assoc.* 2003 Apr;95(4):257–62.

Frassetto LA, Morris RC Jr., Sebastian A. Effect of age on blood acid-base composition in adult humans: role of age-related renal functional decline. *Am J Physiol.* 1996 Dec;271(6 Pt 2):F1114–22.

Frassetto LA, Morris RC Jr., Sellmeyer DE, Todd K, Sebastian A. Diet, evolution, and aging—the pathophysiologic effects of the post-agricultural inversion of the potassium-to-sodium and base-to-chloride ratios in the human diet. *Eur J Nutr.* 2001 Oct;40(5):200–13.

Frassetto LA, Todd KM, Morris RC Jr., Sebastian A. Worldwide incidence of hip fracture in elderly women: relation to consumption of animal and vegetable foods. *J Gerontol A Biol Sci Med Sci.* 2000 Oct;55(10):M585–92.

Freedman BI, Wagenknecht LE, Hairston KG, Bowden DW, Carr JJ, Hightower RC, Gordon EJ, Xu J, Langefeld CD, Divers J. Vitamin D, adiposity, and calcified atherosclerotic plaque in African-Americans. *J Clin Endocrinol Metab.* 2010;95:1076–83.

Froicu M, Weaver V, Wynn TA, McDowell MA, Welsh JE, Cantorna MT. A crucial role for the vitamin D receptor in experimental inflammatory bowel diseases. *Mol Endocrinol.* 2003 Dec;17(12):2386–92. Epub 2003 Sep 18.

Fromm L, Heath DL, Vink R, Nimmo AJ. Magnesium attenuates posttraumatic depression/anxiety following diffuse traumatic brain injury in rats. *J Am Coll Nutr.* 2004 Oct;23(5):529S–533S.

Fronczak CM, Baron AE, Chase HP, Ross C, Brady HL, Hoffman M, Eisenbarth GS, Rewers M, Norris JM. In utero dietary exposures and risk of islet autoimmunity in children. *Diabetes Care.* 2003 Dec;26(12):3237–42.

Gallagher RP, Spinelli JJ, Lee TK. Tanning beds, sunlamps, and risk of cutaneous malignant melanoma. *Cancer Epidemiol Biomarkers Prev.* 2005 Mar;14(3):562–6.

Ganji V, Zhang X, Shaikh N, Tangpricha V. Serum 25-hydroxyvitamin D concentrations are associated with prevalence of metabolic syndrome and various cardiometabolic risk factors in US children and adolescents based on assay-adjusted serum 25-hydroxyvitamin D data from NHANES 2001–2006. *Am J Clin Nutr.* 2011 Jul;94(1):225–33.

Garcion E, Wion-Barbot N, Montero-Menei CN, Berger F, Wion D. New clues about vitamin D functions in the nervous system. *Trends Endocrinol Metab.* 2002 Apr;13(3):100–5.

Garland CF, Comstock GW, Garland FC, Helsing KJ, Shaw EK, Gorham ED. Serum 25-hydroxyvitamin D and colon cancer: eight-year prospective study. *Lancet.* 1989 Nov 18;2(8673):1176–8.

Garland CF, Garland FC, Gorham ED. Epidemiologic evidence for different roles of ultraviolet A and B radiation in melanoma mortality rates. *Ann Epidemiol.* 2003 Jul;13(6):395–404.

Garland CF, Gorham ED, Mohr SB, Grant WB, Giovannucci EL, Lipkin M, Newmark H, Holick MF, Garland FC. Vitamin D and prevention of breast cancer: pooled analysis. *J Steroid Biochem Mol Biol.* 2007 Mar;103(3–5): 708–11.

Garland FC, White MR, Garland CF, Shaw E, Gorham ED. Occupational sunlight exposure and melanoma in the U.S. Navy. *Arch Environ Health.* 1990 Sep–Oct;45(5):261–7.

Gauzzi MC, Purificato C, Donato K, Jin Y, Wang L, Daniel KC, Maghazachi AA, Belardelli F, Adorini L, Gessani S. Suppressive effect of 1-alpha, 25-dihydroxyvitamin D_3 on type I IFN-mediated monocyte differentiation into dendritic cells: impairment of functional activities and chemotaxis. *J Immunol.* 2005 Jan 1;174(1):270–6.

Getzenberg RH, Light BW, Lapco PE, Konety BR, Nangia AK, Acierno JS, Dhir R, et al. Vitamin D inhibition of prostate adenocarcinoma growth and metastasis in the Dunning rat prostate model system. *Urology.* 1997 Dec;50(6):999–1006.

Gilbert R, Martin RM, Beynon R, Harris R, Savovic J, Zuccolo L, Bekkering GE, Fraser WD, Sterne JA, Metcalfe C. Associations of circulating and dietary vitamin

D with prostate cancer risk: a systematic review and dose-response meta-analysis. *Cancer Causes Control.* 2011 Mar;22(3):319–40.

Ginde AA, Scragg R, Schwartz RS, Camargo CA, Jr. Prospective study of serum 25-hydroxyvitamin D level, cardiovascular disease mortality, and all-cause mortality in older U.S. Adults. *J Am Geriatr Soc.* 2009;57:1595–1603.

Ginde AA, Wolfe P, Camargo CA Jr., Schwartz RS. Defining vitamin D status by secondary hyperparathyroidism in the U.S. population. *J Endocrinol Invest.* 2011 May 23. [Epub ahead of print.]

Giovannucci E. The epidemiology of vitamin D and cancer incidence and mortality: a review (United States). *Cancer Causes Control.* 2005 Mar;16(2):83–95.

Giovannucci E, Liu Y, Hollis BW, Rimm EB. 25-hydroxyvitamin D and risk of myocardial infarction in men: a prospective study. *Arch Intern Med.* 2008;168:1174–80.

Giovannucci E, Liu Y, Rimm E et al. Prospective study of predictors of vitamin D status and cancer incidence and mortality in men. *J Nat Cancer Inst.* 2006;5:451–9.

Giovannucci E, Liu Y, Willett WC. Cancer incidence and mortality and vitamin D in black and white male health professionals. *Cancer Epidemiol Biomarkers Prev.* 2006 Dec;15(12):2467–72.

Gloth FM 3rd, Alam W, Hollis B. Vitamin D vs broad spectrum phototherapy in the treatment of seasonal affective disorder. *J Nutr Health Aging.* 1999;3(1):5–7.

Gluckman PD, Hanson MA, Buklijas T, Low FM, Beedle AS. Epigenetic mechanisms that underpin metabolic and cardiovascular diseases. *Nat Rev Endocrinol.* 2009;5(7):401–8.

Godfrey KM, Barker DJ. Fetal nutrition and adult disease. *Am J Clin Nutr.* 2000 May;71(5 Suppl):1344S–52S.

Goldacre MJ, Seagroatt V, Yeates D, Acheson ED. Skin cancer in people with multiple sclerosis: a record linkage study. *J Epidemiol Community Health.* 2004 Feb;58(2):142–4.

Gombart AF, Borregaard N, Koeffler HP. Human cathelicidin antimicrobial peptide (CAMP) gene is a direct target of the vitamin D receptor and is strongly up-regulated in myeloid cells by 1,25-dihydroxyvitamin D_3. *FASEB J.* 2005 Jul;19(9):1067–77.

Gordon CM, DePeter KC, Feldman HA, Grace E, Emans SJ. Prevalence of vitamin D deficiency among healthy adolescents. *Arch Pediatr Adolesc Med.* 2004 Jun;158(6):531–7.

Gorham ED, Garland CF, Garland FC, Grant WB, Mohr SB, Lipkin M, Newmark HL, Giovannucci E, Wei M, Holick MF. Optimal vitamin D status for colorectal cancer prevention: a quantitative meta analysis. *Am J Prev Med.* 2007 Mar;32(3):210–6.

Goswami R, Gupta N, Goswami D, Marwaha RK, Tandon N, Kochupillai N. Prevalence and significance of low 25-hydroxyvitamin D concentrations in healthy subjects in Delhi. *Am J Clin Nutr.* 2000 Aug;72(2):472–5.

Grant WB. An ecological study of cancer incidence and mortality rates in France with respect to latitude, an index for vitamin D production. *Dermatoendocrinol.* 2010 Apr;2(2):62–7.

———. An estimate of premature cancer mortality in the U.S. due to inadequate doses of solar ultraviolet-B radiation. *Cancer.* 2002 Mar 15;94(6):1867–75.

———. Ecologic studies of solar UV-B radiation and cancer mortality rates. *Recent Results Cancer Res.* 2003;164:371–7.

Grant WB. How strong is the evidence that solar ultraviolet B and vitamin D reduce the risk of cancer? An examination using Hill's criteria for causality. *Dermatoendocrinol.* 2009 Jan;1(1):17–24.

Grau MV, Baron JA, Sandler RS, Haile RW, Beach ML, Church TR, Heber D. Vitamin D, calcium supplementation, and colorectal adenomas: results of a randomized trial. *J Natl Cancer Inst.* 2003 Dec 3;95(23):1765–71.

Grazzi L, Andrasik F, Usai S, Bussone G. Magnesium as a treatment for paediatric tension-type headache: a clinical replication series. *Neurol Sci.* 2005 Feb;25(6):338–41.

Gregori S, Giarratana N, Smiroldo S, Uskokovic M, Adorini L. A 1-alpha, 25-dihydroxyvitamin D_3 analog enhances regulatory T-cells and arrests autoimmune diabetes in NOD mice. *Diabetes.* 2002 May;51(5):1367–74.

Griffin MD, Lutz W, Phan VA, Bachman LA, McKean DJ, Kumar R. Dendritic cell modulation by 1-alpha, 25-dihydroxyvitamin D_3 and its analogs: a vitamin D receptor-dependent pathway that promotes a persistent state of immaturity in vitro and in vivo. *Proc Natl Acad Sci USA.* 2001 Jun 5; 98(12):6800–5. Epub 2001 May 22.

Grimaldi CM. Sex and systemic lupus erythematosus: the role of the sex hormones estrogen and prolactin on the regulation of autoreactive B cells. *Curr Opin Rheumatol.* 2006 Sep;18(5):456–61.

Guarner F. Enteric flora in health and disease. *Digestion.* 2006;73 Suppl 1:5–12. Epub 2006 Feb 8.

Guerrero-Romero F, Rodriguez-Moran M. Hypomagnesemia is linked to low serum HDL-cholesterol irrespective of serum glucose values. *J Diabetes Complications.* 2000 Sep–Oct;14(5):272–6.

———. Relationship between serum magnesium levels and C-reactive protein concentration, in non-diabetic, non-hypertensive obese subjects. *Int J Obes Relat Metab Disord.* 2002 Apr;26(4):469–74.

Guerrero-Romero F, Tamez-Perez HE, Gonzalez-Gonzalez G, Salinas-Martinez AM, Montes-Villarreal J, Trevino-Ortiz JH, Rodriguez-Moran M. Oral magnesium supplementation improves insulin sensitivity in non-diabetic subjects with insulin resistance: a double-blind placebo-controlled randomized trial. *Diabetes Metab.* 2004 Jun;30(3):253–8.

Gulseth HL, Gjelstad IM, Tierney AC, Lovegrove JA, Defoort C, Blaak EE, Lopez-Miranda J, Kiec-Wilk B, Ris U, Roche HM, Drevon CA, Birkeland KI. Serum vitamin D concentration does not predict insulin action or secretion in European subjects with the metabolic syndrome. *Diabetes Care.* 2010;33:923–5.

Gurlek A, Pittelkow MR, Kumar R. Modulation of growth factor/cytokine synthesis and signaling by 1-alpha, 25-dihydroxyvitamin D_3: implications in cell growth and differentiation. *Endocr Rev.* 2002 Dec;23(6):763–86.

Haag M, Dippenaar NG. Dietary fats, fatty acids and insulin resistance: short review of a multifaceted connection. *Med Sci Monit.* 2005 Dec;11(12): RA359–67.

Hahn S, Haselhorst U, Tan S, Quadbeck B, Schmidt M, Roesler S, Kimmig R, Mann K, Janssen OE. Low-serum 25-hydroxyvitamin D concentrations are associated with insulin resistance and obesity in women with polycystic ovary syndrome. *Exp Clin Endocrinol Diabetes.* 2006 Nov;114(10): 577–83.

Halton TL, Hu FB. The effects of high-protein diets on thermogenesis, satiety, and weight loss: a critical review. *J Am Coll Nutr.* 2004 Oct;23(5): 373–85.

Hanchette CL, Schwartz GG. Geographic patterns of prostate cancer mortality. Evidence for a protective effect of ultraviolet radiation. *Cancer.* 1992 Dec 15;70(12):2861–9.

Haque WA, Garg A. Adipocyte biology and adipocytokines. *Clin Lab Med.* 2004 Mar;24(1):217–34.

Harris RA, Pedersen-White J, Guo DH, Stallmann-Jorgensen IS, Keeton D, Huang Y, Shah Y, Zhu H, Dong Y. Vitamin D(3) supplementation for 16 weeks improves flow-mediated dilation in overweight African American adults. *Am J Hypertens.* 2011 May;24(5):557–62.

Harris SS, Dawson-Hughes B. Seasonal changes in plasma 25-hydroxyvitamin D concentrations of young American black and white women. *Am J Clin Nutr.* 1998 Jun;67(6):1232–6.

Harris SS, Soteriades E, Dawson-Hughes B; Framingham Heart Study; Boston Low-Income Elderly Osteoporosis Study. Secondary hyperparathyroidism and bone turnover in elderly blacks and whites. *J Clin Endocrinol Metab.* 2001 Aug;86(8):3801–4.

Hashemipour S, Larijani B, Adibi H, Javadi E, Sedaghat M, Pajouhi M, Soltani A, Shafaei AR, Hamidi Z, Fard AR, Hossein-Nezhad A, Booya F. Vitamin D deficiency and causative factors in the population of Tehran. *BMC Public Health.* 2004 Aug 25;4:38.

Haug CJ, Aukrust P, Haug E, Morkrid L, Muller F, Froland SS. Severe deficiency of 1,25-dihydroxyvitamin D_3 in human immunodeficiency virus infection: association with immunological hyperactivity and only minor changes in calcium homeostasis. *J Clin Endocrinol Metab.* 1998 Nov;83(11): 3832–8.

Hayes CE, Cantorna MT, DeLuca HF. Vitamin D and multiple sclerosis. *Proc Soc Exp Biol Med.* 1997 Oct;216(1):21–7.

Hayes CE, Nashold FE, Spach KM, Pedersen LB. The immunological functions of the vitamin D endocrine system. *Cell Mol Biol (Noisy-le-grand).* 2003 Mar;49(2):277–300.

He K, Liu K, Daviglus ML, Morris SJ, Loria CM, Van Horn L, Jacobs DR Jr., Savage PJ. Magnesium intake and incidence of metabolic syndrome among young adults. *Circulation.* 2006 Apr 4;113(13):1675–82.

Heaney RP. Constructive interactions among nutrients and bone-active pharmacologic agents with principal emphasis on calcium, phosphorus, vitamin D, and protein. *J Am Coll Nutr.* 2001 Oct;20(5 Suppl):403S–409S; discussion 417S–420S.

Heaney RP, Barger-Lux MJ, Dowell MS, Chen TC, Holick MF. Calcium absorptive effects of vitamin D and its major metabolites. *J Clin Endocrinol Metab.* 1997 Dec;82(12):4111–6.

Heaney RP, Davies KM, Chen TC, Holick MF, Barger-Lux MJ. Human serum 25-hydroxycholecalciferol response to extended oral dosing with cholecalciferol. *Am J Clin Nutr.* 2003 Jan;77(1):204–10.

Heaney RP, Dowell MS, Hale CA, Bendich A. Calcium absorption varies within the reference range for serum 25-hydroxyvitamin D. *J Am Coll Nutr.* 2003 Apr;22(2):142–6.

Heaney RP, Weaver CM. Calcium absorption from kale. *Am J Clin Nutr.* 1990 Apr;51(4):656–7.

Held K, Antonijevic IA, Kunzel H, Uhr M, Wetter TC, Golly IC, Steiger A, Murck H. Oral Mg(2+) supplementation reverses age-related neuroendocrine and sleep EEG changes in humans. *Pharmacopsychiatry.* 2002 Jul;35(4):135–43.

Helland IB, Smith L, Saarem K, Saugstad OD, Drevon CA. Maternal supplementation with very-long-chain n-3 fatty acids during pregnancy and lactation augments children's IQ at 4 years of age. *Pediatrics.* 2003 Jan;111(1): e39–44.

Henry HL, Bouillon R, Norman AW, Gallagher JC, Lips P, Heaney RP, Vieth R, Pettifor JM, Dawson-Hughes B, Lamberg-Allardt CJ, Ebeling PR. 14th Vitamin D Workshop consensus on vitamin D nutritional guidelines. *J Steroid Biochem Mol Biol.* 2010 Jul;121(1–2):4–6.

Hewison M, Freeman L, Hughes SV, Evans KN, Bland R, Eliopoulos AG, Kilby MD, Moss PA, Chakraverty R. Differential regulation of vitamin D receptor and its ligand in human monocyte-derived dendritic cells. *J Immunol.* 2003 Jun 1;170(11):5382–90.

Hilakivi-Clarke L, Forsen T, Eriksson JG, Luoto R, Tuomilehto J, Osmond C, Barker DJ. Tallness and overweight during childhood have opposing effects on breast cancer risk. *Br J Cancer.* 2001 Nov 30;85(11):1680–4.

Hodgkinson JE, Davidson CL, Beresford J, Sharpe PT. Expression of a human homeobox-containing gene is regulated by 1,25(OH)2D$_3$ in bone cells. *Biochim Biophys Acta.* 1993 Jul 18;1174(1):11–6.

Hoecker CC, Kanegaye JT. First-place winner. Recurrent febrile seizures: an unusual presentation of nutritional rickets. *J Emerg Med.* 2002 Nov;23(4): 367–70.

Holick MF. Vitamin D deficiency. *N Engl J Med.* 2007 Jul 19;357(3):266–81.

Holick MF, Biancuzzo RM, Chen TC, Klein EK, Young A, Bibuld D, Reitz R, Salameh W, Ameri A, Tannenbaum AD. Vitamin D2 is as effective as vitamin D3 in maintaining circulating concentrations of 25-hydroxyvitamin D. *J Clin Endocrinol Metab.* 2008;93:677–81.

Holick MF, Binkley NC, Bischoff-Ferrari HA, Gordon CM, Hanley DA, Heaney RP, Hughes G, Clark E. Regulation of dendritic cells by female sex steroids: relevance to immunity and autoimmunity. *Autoimmunity.* 2007;40(6):470–81.

Holick MF, Binkley NC, Bischoff-Ferrari HA, Gordon CM, Hanley DA, Heaney RP, Murad MH, Weaver CM. Evaluation, treatment, and prevention of vitamin D deficiency: an Endocrine Society clinical practice guideline. *J Clin Ednocrinol Metab.* 2011 Jul;96(7):1911–30.

Holick MF, Smith E, Pincus S. Skin as the site of vitamin D synthesis and target tissue for 1,25-dihydroxyvitamin D$_3$. Use of calcitriol (1,25-dihydroxyvitamin D$_3$) for treatment of psoriasis. *Arch Dermatol.* 1987 Dec;123(12):1677–1683a.

Hollis BW. Editorial: The determination of circulating 25-hydroxyvitamin D: no easy task. *J Clin Endocrinol Metab.* 2004 Jul;89(7):3149–51.

Hollis BW, Wagner CL. Vitamin D requirements during lactation: high-dose maternal supplementation as therapy to prevent hypovitaminosis D for both the mother and the nursing infant. *Am J Clin Nutr.* 2004 Dec;80(6 Suppl):1752S–1758S.

Hooper L, Thompson RL, Harrison RA, Summerbell CD, Ness AR, Moore HJ, Worthington HV, et al. Risks and benefits of omega-3 fats for mortality, cardiovascular disease, and cancer: systematic review. *BMJ.* 2006 Apr 1; 332(7544):752–60. Epub 2006 Mar 24.

Hu FB, Manson JE, Willett WC. Types of dietary fat and risk of coronary heart disease: a critical review. *J Am Coll Nutr.* 2001 Feb;20(1):5–19.

Huerta MG, Roemmich JN, Kington ML, Bovbjerg VE, Weltman AL, Holmes VF, Patrie JT, Rogol AD, Nadler JL. Magnesium deficiency is associated with insulin resistance in obese children. *Diabetes Care.* 2005 May;28(5): 1175–81.

Hughes AM, Armstrong BK, Vajdic CM, Turner J, Grulich AE, Fritschi L, Milliken S, Kaldor J, Benke G, Kricker A. Sun exposure may protect against non-Hodgkin lymphoma: a case-control study. *Int J Cancer.* 2004 Dec 10;112(5): 865–71.

Huisman AM, White KP, Algra A, Harth M, Vieth R, Jacobs JW, Bijlsma JW, Bell DA. Vitamin D levels in women with systemic lupus erythematosus and fibromyalgia. *J Rheumatol.* 2001 Nov;28(11):2535–9.

Humayun MA, Elango R, Ball RO, Pencharz PB. Reevaluation of the protein requirement in young men with the indicator amino acid oxidation technique. *Am J Clin Nutr.* 2007 Oct;86(4):995–1002.

Hunter DJ, Hart D, Snieder H, Bettica P, Swaminathan R, Spector TD. Evidence of altered bone turnover, vitamin D and calcium regulation with knee osteoarthritis in female twins. *Rheumatology (Oxford).* 2003 Nov;42(11): 1311–6. Epub 2003 Jul 16.

Hunter DJ, Spector TD. The role of bone metabolism in osteoarthritis. *Curr Rheumatol Rep.* 2003 Feb;5(1):15–9.

Hutchinson MS, Grimnes G, Joakimsen RM, Figenschau Y, Jorde R. Low serum 25-hydroxyvitamin D levels are associated with increased all-cause mortality risk in a general population: the Tromsø study. *Eur J Endocrinol.* 2010 May;162(5):935–42.

Hypponen E, Laara E, Reunanen A, Jarvelin MR, Virtanen SM. Intake of vitamin D and risk of type 1 diabetes: a birth-cohort study. *Lancet.* 2001 Nov 3;358(9292):1500–3.

Itoh K, Kawasaka T, Nakamura M. The effects of high oral magnesium supplementation on blood pressure, serum lipids and related variables in apparently healthy Japanese subjects. *Br J Nutr.* 1997 Nov;78(5):737–50.

International MHC and Autoimmunity Genetics Network (IMAGEN). Mapping of multiple susceptibility variants within the MHC region of 7 immune-mediated diseases. *PNAS.* 2009;106(44):18680–5.

Jacobs ET, Giuliano AR, Martinez ME, Hollis BW, Reid ME, Marshall JR. Plasma levels of 25-hydroxyvitamin D, 1,25-dihydroxyvitamin D and the risk of prostate cancer. *J Steroid Biochem Mol Biol.* 2004 May; 89–90(1–5):533–7.

Jamerson KA. The disproportionate impact of hypertensive cardiovascular disease in African Americans: getting to the heart of the issue. *J Clin Hypertens (Greenwich).* 2004 Apr;6(4 Suppl 1):4–10.

Janssen HC, Samson MM, Verhaar HJ. Vitamin D deficiency, muscle function, and falls in elderly people. *Am J Clin Nutr.* 2002 Apr;75(4):611–5.

Javaid MK, Crozier SR, Harvey NC, Gale CR, Dennison EM, Boucher BJ, Arden NK, Godfrey KM, Cooper C; Princess Anne Hospital Study Group. Maternal vitamin D status during pregnancy and childhood bone mass at age 9 years: a longitudinal study. *Lancet.* 2006 Jan 7;367(9504):36–43.

Jenab M, Bueno-de-Mesquita HB, Ferrari P, et al. Association between prediagnostic circulating vitamin D concentration and risk of colorectal cancer in European populations: a nested case-control study. *BMJ.* 2010 Jan 21;340.

Jiang F, Li P, Fornace AJ Jr., Nicosia SV, Bai W. G2/M arrest by 1,25-dihydroxyvitamin D_3 in ovarian cancer cells mediated through the induction of GADD45 via an exonic enhancer. *J Biol Chem.* 2003 Nov 28;278(48):48030-40. Epub 2003 Sep 23.

Jiang R, Manson JE, Stampfer MJ, Liu S, Willett WC, Hu FB. Nut and peanut butter consumption and risk of type 2 diabetes in women. *JAMA.* 2002 Nov 27;288(20):2554–60.

John EM, Schwartz GG, Dreon DM, Koo J. Vitamin D and breast cancer risk: the NHANES I Epidemiologic follow-up study, 1971–1975 to 1992. National Health and Nutrition Examination Survey. *Cancer Epidemiol Biomarkers Prev.* 1999 May;8(5):399–406.

Johnston CS, Tjonn SL, Swan PD. High-protein, low-fat diets are effective for weight loss and favorably alter biomarkers in healthy adults. *J Nutr.* 2004 Mar;134(3):586–91.

Jones G. Pharmacokinetics of vitamin D toxicity. *Am J Clin Nutr.* 2008;88:582S–586S.

Jorde R, Bonaa KH. Calcium from dairy products, vitamin D intake, and blood pressure: the Tromso Study. *Am J Clin Nutr.* 2000 Jun;71(6):1530–5.

Jorde R, Figenschau Y. Supplementation with cholecalciferol does not improve glycemic control in diabetic subjects with normal serum 25-hydroxyvitamin D levels. *Eur J Nutr.* 2009;48:349–54.

Jorde R, Haug E, Figenschau Y, Hansen JB. Serum levels of vitamin D and haemostatic factors in healthy subjects: the Tromsø study. *Acta Haematol.* 2006 Nov 28;117(2):91–97.

Jorde R, Sneve M, Hutchinson M, Emaus N, Figenschau Y, Grimnes G. Tracking of serum 25-hydroxyvitamin D levels during 14 years in a population-based study and during 12 months in an intervention study. *Am J Epidemiol.* 2010;171:903–8.

Jorde R, Sundsfjord J, Haug E, Bonaa KH. Relation between low calcium intake, parathyroid hormone, and blood pressure. *Hypertension.* 2000 May;35(5):1154–9.

Jorde R, Waterloo K, Saleh F, Haug E, Svartberg J. Neuropsychological function in relation to serum parathyroid hormone and serum 25-hydroxyvitamin D levels: the Tromsø study. *J Neurol.* 2006 Apr;253(4):464–70. Epub 2005 Nov 14.

Kalhoff H, Manz F. Nutrition, acid-base status and growth in early childhood. *Eur J Nutr.* 2001 Oct;40(5):221–30.

Kalueff AV, Minasyan A, Tuohimaa P. Anticonvulsant effects of 1,25-dihydroxy vitamin D in chemically induced seizures in mice. *Brain Res Bull.* 2005 Sep 30;67(1–2):156–60.

Kalueff AV, Tuohimaa P. Neurosteroid hormone vitamin D and its utility in clinical nutrition. *Curr Opin Clin Nutr Metab Care.* 2007 Jan;10(1):12–9.

Kamen DL, Cooper GS, Bouali H, Shaftman SR, Hollis BW, Gilkeson GS. Vitamin D deficiency in systemic lupus erythematosus. *Autoimmun Rev.* 2006 Feb;5(2):114–7.

Kamycheva E, Joakimsen RM, Jorde R. Intakes of calcium and vitamin D predict body mass index in the population of Northern Norway. *J Nutr.* 2003 Jan;133(1):102–6.

Kantarci O, Wingerchuk D. Epidemiology and natural history of multiple sclerosis: new insights. *Curr Opin Neurol.* 2006 Jun;19(3):248–54.

Kawano Y, Matsuoka H, Takishita S, Omae T. Effects of magnesium supplementation in hypertensive patients: assessment by office, home, and ambulatory blood pressures. *Hypertension.* 1998 Aug;32(2):260–5.

Kawasaki T, Itoh K, Kawasaki M. Reduction in blood pressure with a sodium-reduced, potassium- and magnesium-enriched mineral salt in subjects with mild essential hypertension. *Hypertens Res.* 1998 Dec;21(4):235–43.

Kawashima H, Kraut JA, Kurokawa K. Metabolic acidosis suppresses 25-hydroxyvitamin in D_3-1alpha-hydroxylase in the rat kidney. Distinct site and mechanism of action. *J Clin Invest.* 1982 Jul;70(1):135–40.

Kayaniyil S, Vieth R, Harris SB, Retnakaran R, Knight JA, Gerstein HC, Perkins BA, Zinman B, Hanley AJ. Association of 25(OH)D and PTH with metabolic syndrome and its traditional and nontraditional components. *J Clin Endocrinol Metab.* 2011;96(1):168–75.

Kayaniyil S, Vieth R, Retnakaran R, Knight JA, Qi Y, Gerstein HC, Perkins B, Harris SB, Zinman B, Hanley AJ. Association of vitamin D with insulin resistance and beta-cell dysfunction in subjects at risk for type 2 diabetes. *Diabetes Care.* 2010; Jun;33(6):1379–81.

Kellum JA, Song M, Li J. Science review: extracellular acidosis and the immune response: clinical and physiologic implications. *Crit Care.* 2004 Oct;8(5): 331–6.

Kendrick J, Targher G, Smits G, Chonchol M. 25-hydroxyvitamin D deficiency is independently associated with cardiovascular disease in the Third National Health and Nutrition Examination Survey. *Atherosclerosis.* 2009;205:255–60.

Kenny AM, Mangano KM, Abourizk RH, Bruno RS, Anamani DE, Kleppinger A, Walsh SJ, Prestwood KM, Kerstetter JE. Soy proteins and isoflavones affect bone mineral density in older women: a randomized controlled trial. *Am J Clin Nutr.* 2009 Jul;90(1):234–42.

Kerstetter JE, O'Brien KO, Insogna KL. Dietary protein, calcium metabolism, and skeletal homeostasis revisited. *Am J Clin Nutr.* 2003 Sep;78(3 Suppl): 584S–592S.

Kerstetter JE, Svastisalee CM, Caseria DM, Mitnick ME, Insogna KL. A threshold for low-protein-diet-induced elevations in parathyroid hormone. *Am J Clin Nutr.* 2000 Jul;72(1):168–73.

Kilkkinen A, Knekt P, Aro A, Rissanen H, Marniemi J, Heliovaara M, Impivaara O, Reunanen A. Vitamin D status and the risk of cardiovascular disease death. *Am J Epidemiol.* 2009;170:1032–9.

Kim MK, Il Kang M, Won Oh K, Kwon HS, Lee JH, Lee WC, Yoon KH, Son HY. The association of serum vitamin D level with presence of metabolic syndrome and hypertension in middle-aged Korean subjects. *Clin Endocrinol (Oxf).* 2010 Sep;73(3):330–8.

Kimlin MG, Schallhorn KA. Estimations of the human "vitamin D" UV exposure in the USA. *Photochem Photobiol Sci.* 2004 Nov-Dec;3(11-12):1067–70.

Kiraly SJ, Kiraly MA, Hawe RD, Makhani N. Vitamin D as a neuroactive substance: review. *ScientificWorldJournal.* 2006 Jan 26;6:125–39.

Knutsen KV, Brekke M, Gjelstad S, Lagerløv P. Vitamin D status in patients with musculoskeletal pain, fatigue and headache: a cross-sectional descriptive study in a multi-ethnic general practice in Norway. *Scand J Prim Health Care.* 2010 Sep;28(3):166–71.

Ko P, Burkert R, McGrath J, Eyles D. Maternal vitamin D_3 deprivation and the regulation of apoptosis and cell cycle during rat brain development. *Brain Res Dev Brain Res.* 2004 Oct 15;153(1):61–8.

Kong J, Zhang Z, Musch MW, Ning G, Sun J, Hart J, Bissonnette M, Li YC. Novel role of the vitamin D receptor in maintaining the integrity of the intestinal mucosal barrier. *Am J Physiol Gastrointest Liver Physiol.* 2008 Jan;294(1):G208–16.

Kositsawat J, Freeman VL, Gerber BS, Geraci S. Association of A1c levels with vitamin D status in U.S. Adults: data from the National Health and Nutrition Examination Survey. *Diabetes Care.* 2010;33:1236.

Kozielec T, Starobrat-Hermelin B. Assessment of magnesium levels in children with attention deficit hyperactivity disorder (ADHD). *Magnes Res.* 1997 Jun;10(2):143–8.

Krall EA, Wehler C, Garcia RI, Harris SS, Dawson-Hughes B. Calcium and vitamin D supplements reduce tooth loss in the elderly. *Am J Med.* 2001 Oct 15;111(6):452–6.

Kreiter SR, Schwartz RP, Kirkman HN Jr., Charlton PA, Calikoglu AS, Davenport ML. Nutritional rickets in African American breast-fed infants. *J Pediatr.* 2000 Aug;137(2):153–7.

Kremer JM. N-3 fatty acid supplements in rheumatoid arthritis. *Am J Clin Nutr.* 2000 Jan;71(1 Suppl):349S–351S.

Krishnan AV, Feldman D. Molecular pathways mediating the anti-inflammatory effects of calcitriol: implications for prostate cancer chemoprevention and treatment. *Endocr Relat Cancer.* 2010 Jan 29;17(1):R19–R38.

Krishnan AV, Swami S, Feldman D. Vitamin D and breast cancer: inhibition of estrogen synthesis and signaling. *J Steroid Biochem Mol Biol.* 2010 Jul;121(1–2):343–8.

Krishnan AV, Swami S, Peng L, Wang J, Moreno J, Feldman D. Tissue-selective regulation of aromatase expression by calcitriol: implications for breast cancer therapy. *Endocrinology.* 2010 Jan;151(1):32–42.

Kujala UM, Kaprio J, Sarna S, Koskenvuo M. Relationship of leisure-time physical activity and mortality: the Finnish twin cohort. *JAMA.* 1998 Feb 11;279(6):440–4.

Kurtzke JF, Beebe GW, Norman JE Jr. Epidemiology of multiple sclerosis in U.S. veterans: III. Migration and the risk of MS. *Neurology.* 1985 May;35(5): 672–8.

Kurtzke JF, Delasnerie-Laupretre N, Wallin MT. Multiple sclerosis in North African migrants to France. *Acta Neurol Scand.* 1998 Nov;98(5):302–9.

Kurtzke JF, Goldberg ID. Parkinsonism death rates by race, sex, and geography. *Neurology.* 1988 Oct;38(10):1558–61.

Lagunova Z, Porojnicu AC, Lindberg F, Hexeberg S, Moan J. The dependency of vitamin D status on body mass index, gender, age and season. *Anticancer Res.* 2009;29:3713–20.

Lanham SA, Roberts C, Cooper C, Oreffo RO. Intrauterine programming of bone. Part 1: Alteration of the osteogenic environment. *Osteoporos Int.* 2007 Aug 15.

Lansdowne AT, Provost SC. Vitamin D_3 enhances mood in healthy subjects during winter. *Psychopharmacology (Berl).* 1998 Feb;135(4):319–23.

Larkin EK, Gebretsadik T, Koestner N, Newman MS, Liu Z, et al. Agreement of blood spot card measurements of vitamin D Levels with serum, whole blood specimen types and a dietary recall instrument. *PLoS ONE.* 2011;6(1):e16602.

Larson EB, Wang L, Bowen JD, McCormick WC, Teri L, Crane P, Kukull W. Exercise is associated with reduced risk for incident dementia among persons 65 years of age and older. *Ann Intern Med.* 2006 Jan 17;144(2):73–81.

Larsson SC, Bergkvist L, Wolk A. Magnesium intake in relation to risk of colorectal cancer in women. *JAMA.* 2005 Jan 5;293(1):86–9.

Lee DM, Rutter MK, O'Neill TW, Boonen S, Vanderschueren D, Bouillon R, Bartfai G, Casanueva FF, Finn JD, Forti G, Giwercman A, Han TS, Huhtaniemi IT, Kula K, Lean ME, Pendleton N, Punab M, Silman AJ, Wu FC. Vitamin D, parathyroid hormone and the metabolic syndrome in middle-aged and older European men. *Eur J Endocrinol.* 2009;161:947–54.

Lee JH, O'Keefe JH, Lavie CJ, Marchioli R, Harris WS. Omega-3 fatty acids for cardioprotection. *Mayo Clin Proc.* 2008 Mar;83(3):324–32.

Lee P, Greenfield JR, Seibel MJ, Eisman JA, Center JR. Adequacy of vitamin D replacement in severe deficiency is dependent on body mass index. *Am J Med.* 2009;122:1056–60.

Lehtonen-Veromaa MK, Mottonen TT, Nuotio IO, Irjala KM, Leino AE, Viikari JS. Vitamin D and attainment of peak bone mass among peripubertal Finnish girls: a 3-y prospective study. *Am J Clin Nutr.* 2002 Dec;76(6): 1446–53.

Lemann J Jr., Bushinsky DA, Hamm LL. Bone buffering of acid and base in humans. *Am J Physiol Renal Physiol.* 2003 Nov;285(5):F811–32.

Lemire JM. Immunomodulatory role of 1,25-dihydroxyvitamin D$_3$. *J Cell Biochem.* 1992 May;49(1):26–31.

Lemire JM, Archer DC. 1,25-dihydroxyvitamin D$_3$ prevents the in vivo induction of murine experimental autoimmune encephalomyelitis. *J Clin Invest.* 1991 Mar;87(3):1103–7.

Lemire JM, Ince A, Takashima M. 1,25-dihydroxyvitamin D$_3$ attenuates the expression of experimental murine lupus of MRL/l mice. *Autoimmunity.* 1992;12(2):143–8.

Lemon PW. Beyond the zone: protein needs of active individuals. *J Am Coll Nutr.* 2000 Oct;19(5 Suppl):513S–521S.

Lengqvist J, Mata De Urquiza A, Bergman AC, Willson TM, Sjovall J, Perlmann T, Griffiths WJ. Polyunsaturated fatty acids including docosahexaenoic and arachidonic acid bind to the retinoid X receptor alpha ligand-binding domain. *Mol Cell Proteomics.* 2004 Jul;3(7):692–703. Epub 2004 Apr 8.

Leonard BE. The concept of depression as a dysfunction of the immune system. *Curr Immunol Rev.* 2010 Aug;6(3):205–12.

Levis S, Gomez A, Jimenez C, Veras L, Ma F, Lai S, Hollis B, Roos BA. Vitamin D deficiency and seasonal variation in an adult South Florida population. *J Clin Endocrinol Metab.* 2005 Mar;90(3):1557–62. Epub 2005 Jan 5.

Lewis GF, Carpentier A, Adeli K, Giacca A. Disordered fat storage and mobilization in the pathogenesis of insulin resistance and type 2 diabetes. *Endocr Rev.* 2002 Apr;23(2):201–29.

Ley RE, Backhed F, Turnbaugh P, Lozupone CA, Knight RD, Gordon JI. Obesity alters gut microbial ecology. *Proc Natl Acad Sci USA.* 2005 Aug 2;102(31):11070–5. Epub 2005 Jul 20.

Ley RE, Turnbaugh PJ, Klein S, Gordon JI. Microbial ecology: human gut microbes associated with obesity. *Nature.* 2006 Dec 21;444(7122):1022–3.

Li CI, Malone KE, Daling JR. Differences in breast cancer stage, treatment, and survival by race and ethnicity. *Arch Intern Med.* 2003 Jan 13;163(1):49–56.

Li YC, Kong J, Wei M, Chen ZF, Liu SQ, Cao LP. 1,25-dihydroxyvitamin D3 is a negative endocrine regulator of the renin-angiotensin system. *J Clin Invest.* 2002;110:229–38.

Lin PH, Ginty F, Appel LJ, Aickin M, Bohannon A, Garnero P, Barclay D, Svetkey LP. The DASH diet and sodium reduction improve markers of bone turnover and calcium metabolism in adults. *J Nutr.* 2003 Oct;133(10): 3130–6.

Lin R, Amizuka N, Sasaki T, Aarts MM, Ozawa H, Goltzman D, Henderson JE, White JH. 1-alpha,25-dihydroxyvitamin D$_3$ promotes vascularization of the chondro-osseous junction by stimulating expression of vascular endothelial growth factor and matrix metalloproteinase 9. *J Bone Miner Res.* 2002 Sep;17(9):1604–12.

Liu BA, Gordon M, Labranche JM, Murray TM, Vieth R, Shear NH. Seasonal prevalence of vitamin D deficiency in institutionalized older adults. *J Am Geriatr Soc.* 1997 May;45(5):598–603.

Liu E, Meigs JB, Pittas AG, McKeown NM, Economos CD, Booth SL, Jacques PF. Plasma 25-hydroxyvitamin D is associated with markers of the insulin resistant phenotype in nondiabetic adults. *J Nutr.* 2009;139:329–34.

Liu PT, Stenger S, Li H, Wenzel L, Tan BH, Krutzik SR, Ochoa MT, et al. Toll-like receptor triggering of a vitamin D-mediated human antimicrobial response. *Science.* 2006 Mar 24;311(5768):1770–3. Epub 2006 Feb 23.

Liu S, Song Y, Ford ES, Manson JE, Buring JE, Ridker PM. Dietary calcium, vitamin D, and the prevalence of metabolic syndrome in middle-aged and older U.S. women. *Diabetes Care.* 2005 Dec;28(12):2926–32.

Lock K, Pomerleau J, Causer L, Altmann DR, McKee M. The global burden of disease attributable to low consumption of fruit and vegetables: implications for the global strategy on diet. *Bull World Health Organ.* 2005 Feb;83(2):100–8. Epub 2005 Feb 24.

Looker AC, Dawson-Hughes B, Calvo MS, Gunter EW, Sahyoun NR. Serum 25-hydroxyvitamin D status of adolescents and adults in two seasonal subpopulations from NHANES III. *Bone.* 2002 May;30(5):771–7.

Lopez ER, Zwermann O, Segni M, Meyer G, Reincke M, Seissler J, Herwig J, Usadel KH, Badenhoop K. A promoter polymorphism of the CYP27B1 gene is associated with Addison's disease, Hashimoto's thyroiditis, Graves' disease, and type 1 diabetes mellitus in Germans. *Eur J Endocrinol.* 2004 Aug;151(2):193–7.

Lopez-Ridaura R, Willett WC, Rimm EB, Liu S, Stampfer MJ, Manson JE, Hu FB. Magnesium intake and risk of type 2 diabetes in men and women. *Diabetes Care.* 2004 Jan;27(1):134–40.

Lu L, Pan A, Hu FB, Franco OH, Li H, Li X, Yang X, Chen Y, Yu Z, Lin X. Plasma 25-hydroxyvitamin D concentration and metabolic syndrome among middle-aged and elderly Chinese. *Diabetes Care.* 2009; Jul;32(7):1278–83.

Luo C, Wong J, Brown M, Hooper M, Molyneaux L, Yue DK. Hypovitaminosis D in Chinese type 2 diabetes: lack of impact on clinical metabolic status and bio-markers of cellular inflammation. *Diab Vasc Dis Res.* 2009;6:194–9.

Lytle CD, Sagripanti JL. Predicted inactivation of viruses of relevance to biodefense by solar radiation. *J Virol.* 2005 Nov;79(22):14244–52.

Lyu LC, Hsu CY, Yeh CY, Lee MS, Huang SH, Chen CL. A case-control study of the association of diet and obesity with gout in Taiwan. *Am J Clin Nutr.* 2003 Oct;78(4):690–701.

Ma Y, Trump DL, Johnson CS. Vitamin D in combination cancer treatment. *J Cancer.* 2010 Jul 15;1:101–7.

Macdonald HM, New SA, Fraser WD, Campbell MK, Reid DM. Low dietary potassium intakes and high dietary estimates of net endogenous acid production are associated with low bone mineral density in premenopausal women and increased markers of bone resorption in postmenopausal women. *Am J Clin Nutr.* 2005 Apr;81(4):923–33.

Macdonald HM, New SA, Golden MH, Campbell MK, Reid DM. Nutritional associations with bone loss during the menopausal transition: evidence of a beneficial effect of calcium, alcohol, and fruit and vegetable nutrients and of a detrimental effect of fatty acids. *Am J Clin Nutr.* 2004 Jan;79(1): 155–65.

MacLaughlin J, Holick MF. Aging decreases the capacity of human skin to produce vitamin D₃. *J Clin Invest.* 1985 Oct;76(4):1536–8.

Maletic V, Raison CL. Neurobiology of depression, fibromyalgia and neuropathic pain. *Front Biosci.* 2009 Jun 1;14:5291–338.

Mantell DJ, Owens PE, Bundred NJ, Mawer EB, Canfield AE. 1 alpha,25-dihydroxyvitamin D3 inhibits angiogenesis in vitro and in vivo. *Circ. Res.* 2000;87:214–20.

Manz F. History of nutrition and acid-base physiology. *Eur J Nutr.* 2001 Oct;40(5):189–99.

Marshall TA, Stumbo PJ, Warren JJ, Xie XJ. Inadequate nutrient intakes are common and are associated with low diet variety in rural, community-dwelling elderly. *J Nutr.* 2001 Aug;131(8):2192–6.

Martins D, Wolf M, Pan D, Zadshir A, Tareen N, Thadhani R, Felsenfeld A, Levine B, Mehrotra R, Norris K. Prevalence of cardiovascular risk factors and the serum levels of 25-hydroxyvitamin D in the United States: data from the Third National Health and Nutrition Examination Survey. *Arch Intern Med.* 2007 Jun 11;167(11):1159–65.

Matsuoka LY, Ide L, Wortsman J, MacLaughlin JA, Holick MF. Sunscreens suppress cutaneous vitamin D₃ synthesis. *J Clin Endocrinol Metab.* 1987 Jun;64(6): 1165–8.

Mattson MP, Chan SL. Neuronal and glial calcium signaling in Alzheimer's disease. Cell Calcium. 2003 Oct–Nov;34(4–5):385–97.

Maurer M, Riesen W, Muser J, Hulter HN, Krapf R. Neutralization of Western diet inhibits bone resorption independently of K intake and reduces cortisol secretion in humans. *Am J Physiol Renal Physiol.* 2003 Jan;284(1): F32–40. Epub 2002 Sep 24.

Mauskop A, Altura BT, Altura BM. Serum ionized magnesium levels and serum ionized calcium/ionized magnesium ratios in women with menstrual migraine. *Headache.* 2002 Apr;42(4):242–8.

Mauskop A, Altura BT, Cracco RQ, Altura BM. Intravenous magnesium sulfate rapidly alleviates headaches of various types. *Headache.* 1996 Mar;36(3): 154–60.

McAlindon TE, Felson DT, Zhang Y, Hannan MT, Aliabadi P, Weissman B, Rush D, Wilson PW, Jacques P. Relation of dietary intake and serum levels of vitamin D to progression of osteoarthritis of the knee among participants in the Framingham Study. *Ann Intern Med.* 1996 Sep 1;125(5):353–9.

McCann JC, Ames BN. Is there convincing biological or behavioral evidence linking vitamin D deficiency to brain dysfunction? *FASEB J.* 2008 Apr;22(4): 982–1001.

McCormick CC. Passive diffusion does not play a major role in the absorption of dietary calcium in normal adults. *J Nutr.* 2002 Nov;132(11):3428–30.

McCoy H, Kenney MA. Interactions between magnesium and vitamin D: possible implications in the immune system. *Magnes Res.* 1996 Oct;9(3): 185–203.

McGrath JJ, Burne TH, Féron F, Mackay-Sim A, Eyles DW. Developmental vitamin D deficiency and risk of schizophrenia: a 10-year update. *Schizophr Bull.* 2010; Nov;36(6):1073–8.

McGrath JJ, Feron FP, Burne TH, Mackay-Sim A, Eyles DW. Vitamin D$_3$–implications for brain development. *J Steroid Biochem Mol Biol.* 2004 May; 89–90(1–5):557–60.

McInerney-Leo A, Gwinn-Hardy K, Nussbaum RL. Prevalence of Parkinson's disease in populations of African ancestry: a review. *J Natl Med Assoc.* 2004 Jul;96(7):974–9.

McKay JD, McCullough ML, Ziegler RG, et al. Vitamin D receptor polymorphisms and breast cancer risk: results from the National Cancer Institute Breast and Prostate Cancer Cohort Consortium. *Cancer Epidemiol Biomarkers Prev.* 2009 Jan;18(1):297–305.

Meindl S, Rot A, Hoetzenecker W, Kato S, Cross HS, Elbe-Burger A. Vitamin D receptor ablation alters skin architecture and homeostasis of dendritic epidermal T cells. *Br J Dermatol.* 2005 Feb;152(2):231–41.

Menendez C, Lage M, Peino R, Baldelli R, Concheiro P, Dieguez C, Casanueva FF. Retinoic acid and vitamin D$_3$ powerfully inhibit in vitro leptin secretion by human adipose tissue. *J Endocrinol.* 2001 Aug;170(2):425–31.

Merewood A, Mehta SD, Chen TC, Bauchner H, Holick MF. Association between vitamin D deficiency and primary cesarean section. *J Clin Endocrinol Metab.* 2009 Mar;94(3):940–5.

Merlino LA, Curtis J, Mikuls TR, Cerhan JR, Criswell LA, Saag KG; Iowa Women's Health Study. Vitamin D intake is inversely associated with rheumatoid arthritis: results from the Iowa Women's Health Study. *Arthritis Rheum.* 2004 Jan;50(1):72–7.

Meyskens FL Jr., Szabo E. Diet and cancer: the disconnect between epidemiology and randomized clinical trials. *Cancer Epidemiol Biomarkers Prev.* 2005 Jun;14(6):1366–9.

Michelson D, Stratakis C, Hill L, Reynolds J, Galliven E, Chrousos G, Gold P. Bone mineral density in women with depression. *N Engl J Med.* 1996 Oct 17;335(16):1176–81.

Millen AE, Tucker MA, Hartge P, Halpern A, Elder DE, Guerry D 4th, Holly EA, Sagebiel RW, Potischman N. Diet and melanoma in a case-control study. *Cancer Epidemiol Biomarkers Prev.* 2004 Jun;13(6):1042–51.

Miller AH, Maletic V, Raison CL. Inflammation and its discontents: the role of cytokines in the pathophysiology of major depression. *Biol Psychiatry.* 2009 May 1;65(9):732–41.

Mitch WE. Metabolic and clinical consequences of metabolic acidosis. *J Nephrol.* 2006 Mar–Apr;19 Suppl 9:S70–S75.

Mitsuhashi T, Morris RC, Jr., Ives HE. 1,25-dihydroxyvitamin D3 modulates growth of vascular smooth muscle cells. *J Clin Invest.* 1991;87:1889–95.

Molokhia M, McKeigue P. Risk for rheumatic disease in relation to ethnicity and admixture. *Arthritis Res.* 2000;2(2):115–25. Epub 2000 Feb 24.

Mora JR, Iwata M, von Andrian UH. Vitamin effects on the immune system: vitamins A and D take centre stage. *Nat Rev Immunol.* 2008 Sep;8(9):685–98.

Morariu MA, Linden M. Multiple sclerosis in American blacks. *Acta Neurol Scand.* 1980 Sep;62(3):180–7.

Mori TA, Bao DQ, Burke V, Puddey IB, Beilin LJ. Docosahexaenoic acid but not eicosapentaenoic acid lowers ambulatory blood pressure and heart rate in humans. *Hypertension.* 1999 Aug;34(2):253–60.

Mori TA, Bao DQ, Burke V, Puddey IB, Watts GF, Beilin LJ. Dietary fish as a major component of a weight-loss diet: effect on serum lipids, glucose, and insulin metabolism in overweight hypertensive subjects. *Am J Clin Nutr.* 1999 Nov;70(5):817–25.

Morley R, Carlin JB, Pasco JA, Wark JD. Maternal 25-hydroxyvitamin D and parathyroid hormone concentrations and offspring birth size. *J Clin Endocrinol Metab.* 2006 Mar;91(3):906–12. Epub 2005 Dec 13.

Morris MC, Evans DA, Bienias JL, Tangney CC, Bennett DA, Wilson RS, Aggarwal N, Schneider J. Consumption of fish and n-3 fatty acids and risk of incident Alzheimer disease. *Arch Neurol.* 2003 Jul;60(7):940–6.

Mousain-Bosc M, Roche M, Rapin J, Bali JP. Magnesium VitB$_6$ intake reduces central nervous system hyperexcitability in children. *J Am Coll Nutr.* 2004 Oct;23(5):545S–548S.

Mowat AM, Millington OR, Chirdo FG. Anatomical and cellular basis of immunity and tolerance in the intestine. *J Pediatr Gastroenterol Nutr.* 2004 Jun;39 Suppl 3:S723–S724.

Muldoon MF, Mackey RH, Williams KV, Korytkowski MT, Flory JD, Manuck SB. Low central nervous system serotonergic responsivity is associated with the metabolic syndrome and physical inactivity. *J Clin Endocrinol Metab.* 2004 Jan;89(1):266–71.

Munger KL, Levin LI, Hollis BW, Howard NS, Ascherio A. Serum 25-hydroxyvitamin D levels and risk of multiple sclerosis. *JAMA.* 2006 Dec 20;296(23):2832–8.

Munoz KA, Krebs-Smith SM, Ballard-Barbash R, Cleveland LE. Food intakes of U.S. children and adolescents compared with recommendations. *Pediatrics.* 1997 Sep;100(3 Pt 1):323–9.

Mussolino ME, Jonas BS, Looker AC. Depression and bone mineral density in young adults: results from NHANES III. *Psychosom Med.* 2004 Jul–Aug; 66(4):533–7.

Nagpal J, Pande JN, Bhartia A. A double-blind, randomized, placebo-controlled trial of the short-term effect of vitamin D3 supplementation on insulin sensitivity in apparently healthy, middle-aged, centrally obese men. *Diabet Med.* 2009;26:19–27.

Nakaji S, Shimoyama T, Wada S, Sugawara K, Tokunaga S, MacAuley D, Baxter D. No preventive effect of dietary fiber against colon cancer in the Japanese population: a cross-sectional analysis. *Nutr Cancer.* 2003;45(2):156–9.

Nesby-O'Dell S, Scanlon KS, Cogswell ME, Gillespie C, Hollis BW, Looker AC, Allen C, Doughertly C, Gunter EW, Bowman BA. Hypovitaminosis D prevalence and determinants among African American and white women of reproductive age: third National Health and Nutrition Examination Survey, 1988–1994. *Am J Clin Nutr.* 2002 Jul;76(1):187–92.

Nettleton JA, Katz R. n-3 long-chain polyunsaturated fatty acids in type 2 diabetes: a review. *J Am Diet Assoc*. 2005 Mar;105(3):428–40.

Norman AW, Frankel JB, Heldt AM, Grodsky GM. Vitamin D deficiency inhibits pancreatic secretion of insulin. *Science*. 1980 Aug 15;209(4458): 823–5.

O'Connell TD, Berry JE, Jarvis AK, Somerman MJ, Simpson RU. 1,25-dihydroxyvitamin D3 regulation of cardiac myocyte proliferation and hypertrophy. *Am. J. Physiol*. 1997;272:H1751–H1758.

O'Keefe JH Jr., Cordain L. Cardiovascular disease resulting from a diet and lifestyle at odds with our Paleolithic genome: how to become a 21st-century hunter-gatherer. *Mayo Clin Proc*. 2004 Jan;79(1):101–8.

O'Shea J, Paul W. Mechanisms underlying lineage commitment and plasticity of helper CD4+ T Cells. *Science*. 2010; 327(5969): 1098–102.

Oh J, Weng S, Felton SK, Bhandare S, Riek A, Butler B, Proctor BM, Petty M, Chen Z, Schechtman KB, Bernal-Mizrachi L, Bernal-Mizrachi C. 1,25(OH)2 vitamin D inhibits foam cell formation and suppresses macrophage cholesterol uptake in patients with type 2 diabetes mellitus. *Circulation*. 2009;120: 687–98.

Ohkusa T, Nomura T, Sato N. The role of bacterial infection in the pathogenesis of inflammatory bowel disease. *Intern Med*. 2004 Jul;43(7):534–9.

Oosterwerff MM, Eekhoff EM, Heymans MW, Lips P, van Schoor NM. Serum 25-hydroxyvitamin D levels and the metabolic syndrome in older persons. A population-based study. *Clin Endocrinol* (Oxf). 2011 Nov;75(5):608–13. doi: 10.1111/j.1365-265.2011.04110.x.

Osborne JE, Hutchinson PE. Vitamin D and systemic cancer: is this relevant to malignant melanoma? *Br J Dermatol*. 2002 Aug;147(2):197–213.

Owen MJ, O'Donovan MC, Thapar A, Craddock N. Neurodevelopmental hypothesis of schizophrenia. *Br J Psychiatry*. 2011 Mar;198(3):173–5.

Pak CY, Fuller C, Sakhaee K, Preminger GM, Britton F. Long-term treatment of calcium nephrolithiasis with potassium citrate. *J Urol*. 1985 Jul;134(1): 11–9.

Pak CY, Sakhaee K, Moe O, Preminger GM, Poindexter JR, Peterson RD, Pietrow P, Ekeruo W. Biochemical profile of stone-forming patients with diabetes mellitus. *Urology*. 2003 Mar;61(3):523–7.

Parker J, Hashmi O, Dutton D, Mavrodaris A, Stranges S, Kandala NB, Clarke A, Franco OH. Levels of vitamin D and cardiometabolic disorders: systematic review and meta-analysis. *Maturitas*. 2010 Mar;65(3):225–36.

Patel S, Farragher T, Bunn D, et al. Association between serum vitamin D metabolite levels and disease activity in patients with early inflammatory polyarthritis. *Arthritis Rheum*. 2007;56(7): 2143–9.

Pawley N, Bishop NJ. Prenatal and infant predictors of bone health: the influence of vitamin D. *Am J Clin Nutr*. 2004 Dec;80(6 Suppl):1748S–1751S.

Penna G, Adorini L. 1 alpha,25-dihydroxyvitamin D_3 inhibits differentiation, maturation, activation, and survival of dendritic cells leading to impaired alloreactive T-cell activation. *J Immunol*. 2000 Mar 1;164(5):2405–11.

Pettifor JM. Nutritional rickets: deficiency of vitamin D, calcium, or both? *Am J Clin Nutr*. 2004 Dec; 80(6 Suppl):1725S–1729S.

Pfeifer M, Begerow B, Minne HW, Nachtigall D, Hansen C. Effects of a short-term vitamin D_3 and calcium supplementation on blood pressure and parathyroid hormone levels in elderly women. *J Clin Endocrinol Metab.* 2001 Apr;86(4):1633–7.

Pichler J, Gerstmayr M, Szepfalusi Z, Urbanek R, Peterlik M, Willheim M. 1 alpha,25(OH)2D$_3$ inhibits not only Th1 but also Th2 differentiation in human cord blood T-cells. *Pediatr Res.* 2002 Jul;52(1):12–8.

Pilz S, Dobnig H, Nijpels G, Heine RJ, Stehouwer CD, Snijder MB, van Dam RM, Dekker JM. Vitamin D and mortality in older men and women. *Clin Endocrinol* (Oxf). 2009;71:666–72.

Pilz S, Dobnig H, Winklhofer-Roob B et al. Low serum levels of 25-hydroxyvitamin D predict fatal cancer in patients referred to coronary angiography. *Cancer Epidemiology, Biomarkers & Prevention.* 2008;17:1228–33.

Pilz S, Marz W, Wellnitz B, Seelhorst U, Fahrleitner-Pammer A, Dimai HP, Boehm BO, Dobnig H. Association of vitamin D deficiency with heart failure and sudden cardiac death in a large cross-sectional study of patients referred for coronary angiography. *J Clin Endocrinol Metab.* 2008;93:3927–35.

Pinelli NR, Jaber LA, Brown MB, Herman WH. Serum 25-hydroxyvitamin D and insulin resistance, metabolic syndrome, and glucose intolerance among Arab Americans. *Diabetes Care.* 2010; Jun;33(6):1373–5.

Ping-Delfos WC, Soares MJ, Cummings NK. Acute suppression of spontaneous food intake following dairy calcium and vitamin D. *Asia Pac J Clin Nutr.* 2004;13(Suppl):S82.

Pittas AG, Chung M, Trikalinos T, Mitri J, Brendel M, Patel K, Lichtenstein AH, Lau J, Balk EM. Systematic review: vitamin D and cardiometabolic outcomes. *Ann Intern Med.* 2010;152:307–14.

Pittas AG, Harris SS, Stark PC, Dawson-Hughes B. The effects of calcium and vitamin D supplementation on blood glucose and markers of inflammation in nondiabetic adults. *Diabetes Care.* 2007;30:980–6.

Platz EA, Leitzmann MF, Hollis BW, Willett WC, Giovannucci E. Plasma 1, 25-dihydroxy- and 25-hydroxyvitamin D and subsequent risk of prostate cancer. *Cancer Causes Control.* 2004 Apr;15(3):255–65.

Plotnikoff GA, Quigley JM. Prevalence of severe hypovitaminosis D in patients with persistent, nonspecific musculoskeletal pain. *Mayo Clin Proc.* 2003 Dec;78(12):1463–70.

Prabhala A, Garg R, Dandona P. Severe myopathy associated with vitamin D deficiency in western New York. *Arch Intern Med.* 2000 Apr 24;160(8): 1199–203.

Priemel M, von Domarus C, Klatte TO, Kessler S, Schlie J, Meier S, Proksch N, Pastor F, Netter C, Streichert T, Püschel K, Amling M. Bone mineralization defects and vitamin D deficiency: histomorphometric analysis of iliac crest bone biopsies and circulating 25-hydroxyvitamin D in 675 patients. *J Bone Miner Res.* 2010 Feb;25(2):305–12.

Prynne CJ, Ginty F, Paul AA, Bolton-Smith C, Stear SJ, Jones SC, Prentice A. Dietary acid-base balance and intake of bone-related nutrients in Cambridge teenagers. *Eur J Clin Nutr.* 2004 Nov;58(11):1462–71.

Puchacz E, Stumpf WE, Stachowiak EK, Stachowiak MK. Vitamin D increases expression of the tyrosine hydroxylase gene in adrenal medullary cells. *Brain Res Mol Brain Res.* 1996 Feb;36(1):193–6.

Rachdi L, Balcazar N, Elghazi L, Barker DJ, Krits I, Kiyokawa H, Bernal-Mizrachi E. Differential effects of p27 in regulation of beta-cell mass during development, neonatal period, and adult life. *Diabetes.* 2006 Dec;55(12):3520–8.

Rajakumar K. Vitamin D, cod-liver oil, sunlight, and rickets: a historical perspective. *Pediatrics.* 2003 Aug;112(2):e132–5.

Ramagopalan SV, Maugeri NJ, Handunnetthi L, Lincoln MR, Orton SM, Dyment DA, Deluca GC, Herrera BM, Chao MJ, Sadovnick AD, Ebers GC, Knight JC. Expression of the multiple sclerosis-associated MHC class II Allele HLA-DRB1*1501 is regulated by vitamin D. *PLoS Genet.* 2009 Feb;5(2):e1000369.

Ravid A, Rubinstein E, Gamady A, Rotem C, Liberman UA, Koren R. Vitamin D inhibits the activation of stress-activated protein kinases by physiological and environmental stresses in keratinocytes. *J Endocrinol.* 2002 Jun;173(3):525–32.

Reddy ST, Wang CY, Sakhaee K, Brinkley L, Pak CY. Effect of low-carbohydrate high-protein diets on acid-base balance, stone-forming propensity, and calcium metabolism. *Am J Kidney Dis.* 2002 Aug;40(2):265–74.

Reinhardt TA, Stabel JR, Goff JP. 1,25-dihydroxyvitamin D_3 enhances milk antibody titers to *Escherichia coli* J5 vaccine. *J Dairy Sci.* 1999 Sep;82(9): 1904–9.

Remer T. Influence of nutrition on acid-base balance: metabolic aspects. *Eur J Nutr.* 2001 Oct;40(5):214–20.

Remer T, Manz F. Potential renal acid load of foods and its influence on urine pH. *J Am Diet Assoc.* 1995 Jul;95(7):791–7.

Reusser ME, DiRienzo DB, Miller GD, McCarron DA. Adequate nutrient intake can reduce cardiovascular disease risk in African Americans. *J Natl Med Assoc.* 2003 Mar;95(3):188–95.

Rigby WF, Denome S, Fanger MW. Regulation of lymphokine production and human T lymphocyte activation by 1,25-dihydroxyvitamin D_3: specific inhibition at the level of messenger RNA. *J Clin Invest.* 1987 Jun;79(6): 1659–64.

Riggs JE. Neurologic manifestations of electrolyte disturbances. *Neurol Clin.* 2002 Feb;20(1):227–39, vii.

Rizzoli R, Bianchi ML, Garabédian M, McKay HA, Moreno LA. Maximizing bone mineral mass gain during growth for the prevention of fractures in the adolescents and the elderly. *Bone.* 2010 Feb;46(2):294–305.

Rodriguez C, McCullough ML, Mondul AM, Jacobs EJ, Fakhrabadi-Shokoohi D, Giovannucci EL, Thun MJ, Calle EE. Calcium, dairy products, and risk of prostate cancer in a prospective cohort of United States men. *Cancer Epidemiol Biomarkers Prev.* 2003 Jul;12(7):597–603.

Rosanoff A, Seelig MS. Comparison of mechanism and functional effects of magnesium and statin pharmaceuticals. *J Am Coll Nutr.* 2004 Oct;23(5): 501S–505S.

Rosen CJ, Morrison A, Zhou H, Storm D, Hunter SJ, Musgrave K, Chen T, Wei W, Holick MF. Elderly women in northern New England exhibit seasonal changes in bone mineral density and calciotropic hormones. *Bone Miner.* 1994 May;25(2):83–92.

Rostand SG. Ultraviolet light may contribute to geographic and racial blood pressure differences. *Hypertension.* 1997 Aug;30(2 Pt 1):150–6.

Rostand SG, Cliver SP, Goldenberg RL. Racial disparities in the association of foetal growth retardation to childhood blood pressure. *Nephrol Dial Transplant.* 2005 Aug;20(8):1592–7. Epub 2005 Apr 19.

Rucker D, Allan JA, Fick GH, Hanley DA. Vitamin D insufficiency in a population of healthy western Canadians. *CMAJ.* 2002 Jun 11;166(12):1517–24.

Rude RK, Gruber HE. Magnesium deficiency and osteoporosis: animal and human observations. *J Nutr Biochem.* 2004 Dec;15(12):710–6.

Rude RK, Gruber HE, Norton HJ, Wei LY, Frausto A, Kilburn J. Reduction of dietary magnesium by only 50 percent in the rat disrupts bone and mineral metabolism. *Osteoporos Int.* 2006;17(7):1022–32. Epub 2006 Apr 7.

Rude RK, Gruber HE, Norton HJ, Wei LY, Frausto A, Mills BG. Bone loss induced by dietary magnesium reduction to 10 percent of the nutrient requirement in rats is associated with increased release of substance P and tumor necrosis factor-alpha. *J Nutr.* 2004 Jan;134(1):79–85.

Sabate J. Nut consumption, vegetarian diets, ischemic heart disease risk, and all-cause mortality: evidence from epidemiologic studies. *Am J Clin Nutr.* 1999 Sep;70(3 Suppl):500S–503S.

Saleh F, Jorde R, Sundsfjord J, Haug E, Figenschau Y. Causes of secondary hyperparathyroidism in a healthy population: the Tromsø study. *J Bone Miner Metab.* 2006;24(1):58–64.

Samanic C, Gridley G, Chow WH, Lubin J, Hoover RN, Fraumeni JF Jr. Obesity and cancer risk among white and black United States veterans. *Cancer Causes Control.* 2004 Feb;15(1):35–43.

Saris WH, Blair SN, van Baak MA, Eaton SB, Davies PS, Di Pietro L, Fogelholm M, et al. How much physical activity is enough to prevent unhealthy weight gain? Outcome of the IASO 1st Stock Conference and consensus statement. *Obes Rev.* 2003 May;4(2):101–14.

Sato Y, Kikuyama M, Oizumi K. High prevalence of vitamin D deficiency and reduced bone mass in Parkinson's disease. *Neurology.* 1997 Nov;49(5): 1273–8.

Sauvaget C, Nagano J, Allen N, Kodama K. Vegetable and fruit intake and stroke mortality in the Hiroshima/Nagasaki Life Span Study. *Stroke.* 2003 Oct;34(10):2355–60. Epub 2003 Sep 18.

Schleithoff SS, Zittermann A, Tenderich G, Berthold HK, Stehle P, Koerfer R. Vitamin D supplementation improves cytokine profiles in patients with congestive heart failure: a double-blind, randomized, placebo-controlled trial. *Am J Clin Nutr.* 2006 Apr;83(4):754–9.

Schoenberg BS, Osuntokun BO, Adeuja AO, Bademosi O, Nottidge V, Anderson DW, Haerer AF. Comparison of the prevalence of Parkinson's disease in black populations in the rural United States and in rural Nigeria: door-to-door community studies. *Neurology.* 1988 Apr;38(4): 645–6.

Schwartz GG, Oeler TA, Uskokovic MR, Bahnson RR. Human prostate cancer cells: inhibition of proliferation by vitamin D analogs. *Anticancer Res.* 1994 May–Jun;14(3A):1077–81.

Schwartz GG, Wang MH, Zang M, Singh RK, Siegal GP. 1-alpha,25-dihydroxyvitamin D (calcitriol) inhibits the invasiveness of human prostate cancer cells. *Cancer Epidemiol Biomarkers Prev.* 1997 Sep;6(9):727–32.

Schwartz GG, Whitlatch LW, Chen TC, Lokeshwar BL, Holick MF. Human prostate cells synthesize 1,25-dihydroxyvitamin D_3 from 25-hydroxyvitamin D_3. *Cancer Epidemiol Biomarkers Prev.* 1998 May;7(5):391–5.

Scragg RK, Camargo CA, Jr., Simpson RU. Relation of serum 25-hydroxyvitamin D to heart rate and cardiac work (from the National Health and Nutrition Examination Surveys). *Am J Cardiol.* 2010;105:122–8.

Sebastian A, Frassetto LA, Sellmeyer DE, Merriam RL, Morris RC Jr. Estimation of the net acid load of the diet of ancestral preagricultural Homo sapiens and their hominid ancestors. *Am J Clin Nutr.* 2002 Dec;76(6):1308–16.

Sebastian A, Harris ST, Ottaway JH, Todd KM, Morris RC Jr. Improved mineral balance and skeletal metabolism in postmenopausal women treated with potassium bicarbonate. *N Engl J Med.* 1994 Jun 23;330(25):1776–81.

Seifert M, Rech M, Meineke V, Tilgen W, Reichrath J. Differential biological effects of 1,25-dihydroxyvitamin D_3 on melanoma cell lines in vitro. *J Steroid Biochem Mol Biol.* 2004 May;89–90(1–5):375–9.

Sellmeyer DE, Stone KL, Sebastian A, Cummings SR. A high ratio of dietary animal to vegetable protein increases the rate of bone loss and the risk of fracture in postmenopausal women. Study of Osteoporotic Fractures Research Group. *Am J Clin Nutr.* 2001 Jan;73(1):118–22.

Semba RD, Houston DK, Ferrucci L, Cappola AR, Sun K, Guralnik JM, Fried LP. Low serum 25-hydroxyvitamin D concentrations are associated with greater all-cause mortality in older community-dwelling women. *Nutr Res.* 2009;29:525–30.

Sharief S, Jariwala S, Kumar J, Muntner P, Melamed ML. Vitamin D levels and food and environmental allergies in the United States: results from the National Health and Nutrition Examination Survey 2005–2006. *J Allergy Clin Immunol.* 2011;127(5):1195–202.

Sharkey JR, Giuliani C, Haines PS, Branch LG, Busby-Whitehead J, Zohoori N. Summary measure of dietary musculoskeletal nutrient (calcium, vitamin D, magnesium, and phosphorus) intakes is associated with lower-extremity physical performance in homebound elderly men and women. *Am J Clin Nutr.* 2003 Apr;77(4):847–56.

Shikari M, Kushida K, Yamazaki K, Nagai T, Inoue T, Orimo H. Effects of 2 years' treatment of osteoporosis with 1-alpha-hydroxyvitamin D_3 on bone mineral density and incidence of fracture: a placebo-controlled, double-blind prospective study. *Endocr J.* 1996 Apr;43(2):211–20.

Shin MH, Holmes MD, Hankinson SE, Wu K, Colditz GA, Willett WC. Intake of dairy products, calcium, and vitamin D and risk of breast cancer. *J Natl Cancer Inst.* 2002 Sep 4;94(17):1301–11.

Simopoulos AP. The Mediterranean diets: What is so special about the diet of Greece? The scientific evidence. *J Nutr.* 2001 Nov;131(11 Suppl):3065S–73S.

Singh RB. Effect of dietary magnesium supplementation in the prevention of coronary heart disease and sudden cardiac death. *Magnes Trace Elem.* 1990;9(3):143–51.

Sinton LW, Finlay RK, Lynch PA. Sunlight inactivation of fecal bacteriophages and bacteria in sewage-polluted seawater. *Appl Environ Microbiol.* 1999 Aug;65(8):3605–13.

Smedby KE, Hjalgrim H, Melbye M, Torrang A, Rostgaard K, Munksgaard L, Adami J, et al. Ultraviolet radiation exposure and risk of malignant lymphomas. *J Natl Cancer Inst.* 2005 Feb 2;97(3):199–209.

Solomon CC, White E, Kristal AR, Vaughan T. Melanoma and lifetime UV radiation. *Cancer Causes Control.* 2004 Nov;15(9):893–902.

Somjen D, Weisman Y, Kohen F, Gayer B, Limor R, Sharon O, Jaccard N, Knoll E, Stern N. 25-hydroxyvitamin D3-1alpha-hydroxylase is expressed in human vascular smooth muscle cells and is upregulated by parathyroid hormone and estrogenic compounds. *Circulation.* 2005;111(13):1666–71.

Souberbielle JC, Body JJ, Lappe JM, Plebani M, Shoenfeld Y, Wang TJ, Bischoff-Ferrari HA, Cavalier E, Ebeling PR, Fardellone P, Gandini S, Gruson D, Guérin AP, Beickendorff L, Hollis BW, Ish-Shalom S, Jean G, von Landenberg P, Largura A, Olsson T, Pierrot-Deseilligny C, Pilz S, Tincani A, Valcour A, Zittermann A. Vitamin D and musculoskeletal health, cardiovascular disease, autoimmunity and cancer: Recommendations for clinical practice. *Autoimmun Rev.* 2010 Sep;9(11):709–15.

Spach KM, Hayes CE. Vitamin D$_3$ confers protection from autoimmune encephalomyelitis only in female mice. J Immunol. 2005 Sep 15;175(6): 4119–26.

Specker B. Vitamin D requirements during pregnancy. *Am J Clin Nutr.* 2004 Dec;80(6 Suppl):1740S–1747S.

Spence JD. Nutrition and stroke prevention. *Stroke.* 2006 Sep;37(9):2430–5. Epub 2006 Jul 27.

Stagg AJ, Hart AL, Knight SC, Kamm MA. The dendritic cell: its role in intestinal inflammation and relationship with gut bacteria. *Gut.* 2003 Oct;52 (10): 1522–9.

Staples JA, Ponsonby AL, Lim LL, McMichael AJ. Ecologic analysis of some immune-related disorders, including type 1 diabetes, in Australia: latitude, regional ultraviolet radiation, and disease prevalence. *Environ Health Perspect.* 2003 Apr;111(4):518–23.

Starobrat-Hermelin B, Kozielec T. The effects of magnesium physiological supplementation on hyperactivity in children with attention deficit hyperactivity disorder (ADHD): positive response to magnesium oral loading test. *Magnes Res.* 1997 Jun;10(2):149–56.

Stein CJ, Colditz GA. The epidemic of obesity. *J Clin Endocrinol Metab.* 2004 Jun;89(6):2522–5.

Stein EM, Laing EM, Hall DB, Hausman DB, Kimlin MG, Johnson MA, Modlesky CM, Wilson AR, Lewis RD. Serum 25-hydroxyvitamin D concentrations in girls aged 4–8 y living in the southeastern United States. *Am J Clin Nutr.* 2006 Jan;83(1):75–81.

Stene LC, Joner G; Norwegian Childhood Diabetes Study Group. Use of cod-liver oil during the first year of life is associated with lower risk of childhood-onset type 1 diabetes: a large, population-based, case-control study. *Am J Clin Nutr.* 2003 Dec;78(6):1128–34.

Stewart R, Richards M, Brayne C, Mann A. Vascular risk and cognitive impairment in an older, British, African-Caribbean population. *J Am Geriatr Soc.* 2001 Mar;49(3):263–9.

Stumpf WE, Privette TH. Light, vitamin D and psychiatry. Role of 1,25 dihydroxyvitamin D_3 (soltriol) in etiology and therapy of seasonal affective disorder and other mental processes. *Psychopharmacology (Berl).* 1989;97 (3):285–94.

Sun J. Vitamin D and mucosal immune function. *Curr Opin Gastroenterol.* 2010;26(6):591–5.

Sutton AL, MacDonald PN. Vitamin D: more than a "bone-a-fide" hormone. *Mol Endocrinol.* 2003 May;17(5):777–91. Epub 2003 Mar 13.

Switzer KC, McMurray DN, Morris JS, Chapkin RS. (n-3) polyunsaturated fatty acids promote activation-induced cell death in murine T lymphocytes. *J Nutr.* 2003 Feb;133(2):496–503.

Szulc P, Claustrat B, Delmas PD. Serum concentrations of 17beta-e2 and 25- hydroxycholecalciferol 25(OH)D in relation to all-cause mortality in older men—The Minos Study. *Clin Endocrinol* (Oxf). 2009;71:594–602.

Takahashi S, Yamamoto T, Moriwaki Y, Tsutsumi Z, Yamakita J, Higashino K. Decreased serum concentrations of 1,25(OH)2-vitamin D_3 in patients with gout. *Adv Exp Med Biol.* 1998;431:57–60.

Tangpricha V, Pearce EN, Chen TC, Holick MF. Vitamin D insufficiency among free-living healthy young adults. *Am J Med.* 2002 Jun 1;112(8): 659–62.

Tangpricha V, Turner A, Spina C, Decastro S, Chen TC, Holick MF. Tanning is associated with optimal vitamin D status (serum 25-hydroxyvitamin D concentration) and higher bone mineral density. *Am J Clin* Nutr. 2004 Dec;80(6): 1645–9.

Taniura H, Ito M, Sanada N, Kuramoto N, Ohno Y, Nakamichi N, Yoneda Y. Chronic vitamin D_3 treatment protects against neurotoxicity by glutamate in association with upregulation of vitamin D receptor mRNA expression in cultured rat cortical neurons. *J Neurosci Res.* 2006 May 15;83(7): 1179–89.

Targher G, Bertolini L, Padovani R, Zenari L, Scala L, Cigolini M, Arcaro G. Serum 25-hydroxyvitamin D_3 concentrations and carotid artery intima-media thickness among type 2 diabetic patients. *Clin Endocrinol* (Oxf). 2006 Nov;65(5):593–7.

Tetlow LC, Woolley DE. Expression of vitamin D receptors and matrix metalloproteinases in osteoarthritic cartilage and human articular chondrocytes in vitro. *Osteoarthritis Cartilage.* 2001 Jul;9(5):423–31.

Thys-Jacobs S. Alleviation of migraines with therapeutic vitamin D and calcium. *Headache*. 1994 Nov–Dec;34(10):590–2.

Trauninger A, Pfund Z, Koszegi T, Czopf J. Oral magnesium load test in patients with migraine. *Headache*. 2002 Feb;42(2):114–9.

Trivedi DP, Doll R, Khaw KT. Effect of four monthly oral vitamin D_3 (cholecalciferol) supplementation on fractures and mortality in men and women living in the community: randomized double-blind controlled trial. *BMJ*. 2003 Mar 1;326(7387):469.

Turnbaugh PJ, Ley RE, Mahowald MA, Magrini V, Mardis ER, Gordon JI. An obesity-associated gut microbiome with increased capacity for energy harvest. *Nature*. 2006 Dec 21;444(7122):1027–131.

Vaisberg MW, Kaneno R, Franco MF, Mendes NF. Influence of cholecalciferol (vitamin D3) on the course of experimental systemic lupus erythematosus in F1 (NZBxW) mice. *J Clin Lab Anal*. 2000;14(3):91–6.

Vaitkevicius H, Witt R, Maasdam M, Walters K, Gould M, Mackenzie S, Farrow S, Lockette W. Ethnic differences in titratable acid excretion and bone mineralization. *Med Sci Sports Exerc*. 2002 Feb;34(2):295–302.

Valimaki VV, Alfthan H, Lehmuskallio E, Loyttyniemi E, Sahi T, Stenman UH, Suominen H, Valimaki MJ. Vitamin D status as a determinant of peak bone mass in young Finnish men. *J Clin Endocrinol Metab*. 2004 Jan;89(1): 76–80.

Valsamis HA, Arora SK, Labban B, McFarlane SI. Antiepileptic drugs and bone metabolism. *Nutr Metab*. 2006 Sep 6;3:36.

van Wouwe JP, Mattiazzo GF, el Mokadem N, Reeser HM, Hirasing RA. [The incidence and initial symptoms of diabetes mellitus type 1 in 0–14-year-olds in the Netherlands, 1996–1999] *Ned Tijdschr Geneeskd*. 2004 Sep 11;148(37):1824–9.

Vaskonen T. Dietary minerals and modification of cardiovascular risk factors. *J Nutr Biochem*. 2003 Sep;14(9):492–506.

Vassallo M, Camargo C. Potential mechanism for the hypothesized link between sunshine, vitamin D, and food allergy in children. *J Allerg Clin Immunol*. 2010;126:217–22.

Venables MC, Achten J, Jeukendrup AE. Determinants of fat oxidation during exercise in healthy men and women: a cross-sectional study. *J Appl Physiol*. 2005 Jan;98(1):160–7.

Vermeulen ME, Gamberale R, Trevani AS, Martinez D, Ceballos A, Sabatte J, Giordano M, Geffner JR. The impact of extracellular acidosis on dendritic cell function. *Crit Rev Immunol*. 2004;24(5):363–84.

Vermeulen ME, Giordano M, Trevani AS, Sedlik C, Gamberale R, Fernandez-Calotti P, Salamone G, Raiden S, Sanjurjo J, Geffner JR. Acidosis improves uptake of antigens and MHC class I-restricted presentation by dendritic cells. *J Immunol*. 2004 Mar 1;172(5):3196–204.

Viard JP, Souberbielle JC, Kirk O, Reekie J, Knysz B, Losso M, Gatell J, Pedersen C, Bogner JR, Lundgren JD, Mocroft A; for the EuroSIDA Study Group. Vitamin D and clinical disease progression in HIV infection: results from the EuroSIDA study. *AIDS*. 2011 Jun 19; 25(10):1305–15.

Vickers MH, Breier BH, Cutfield WS, Hofman PL, Gluckman PD. Fetal origins of hyperphagia, obesity, and hypertension and postnatal amplification by hyper-caloric nutrition. *Am J Physiol Endocrinol Metab.* 2000 Jul;279(1): E83–7.

Vieth R. Vitamin D supplementation, 25-hydroxyvitamin D concentrations, and safety. *Am J Clin Nutr.* 1999 May;69(5):842–56.

Vieth R, Bischoff-Ferrari H, Boucher BJ, Dawson-Hughes B, Garland CF, Heaney RP, Holick MF, et al. A. The urgent need to recommend an intake of vitamin D that is effective. *Am J Clin Nutr.* 2007 Mar;85(3):649–50.

Vieth R, Chan PC, MacFarlane GD. Efficacy and safety of vitamin D_3 intake exceeding the lowest observed adverse effect level. *Am J Clin Nutr.* 2001 Feb;73(2):288–94.

Vieth R, Kimball S, Hu A, Walfish PG. Randomized comparison of the effects of the vitamin D_3 adequate intake versus 100 mcg (4000 IU) per day on biochemical responses and the well-being of patients. *Nutr J.* 2004 Jul 19;3(1):8.

Visser M, Deeg DJ, Lips P; Longitudinal Aging Study Amsterdam. Low vitamin D and high parathyroid hormone levels as determinants of loss of muscle strength and muscle mass (sarcopenia): the Longitudinal Aging Study Amsterdam. *J Clin Endocrinol Metab.* 2003 Dec;88(12):5766–72.

von Hurst PR, Stonehouse W, Coad J. Vitamin D supplementation reduces insulin resistance in south Asian women living in new Zealand who are insulin resistant and vitamin D deficient—a randomized, placebo-controlled trial. *Br J Nutr.* 2010;103:549–55.

Vormann J, Worlitschek M, Goedecke T, Silver B. Supplementation with alkaline minerals reduces symptoms in patients with chronic low back pain. *J Trace Elem Med Biol.* 2001;15(2–3):179–83.

Walker VP, Modlin RL. The vitamin D connection to pediatric infections and immune function. *Pediatr Res.* 2009 May;65(5 Pt 2):106R–113R.

Wallin MT, Page WF, Kurtzke JF. Multiple sclerosis in U.S. veterans of the Vietnam era and later military service: race, sex, and geography. *Ann Neurol.* 2004 Jan;55(1):65–71.

Wang TJ, Pencina MJ, Booth SL, Jacques PF, Ingelsson E, Lanier K, Benjamin EJ, D'Agostino RB, Wolf M, Vasan RS. Vitamin D deficiency and risk of cardiovascular disease. *Circulation.* 2008;117(4):503–11.

Wang TJ, Zhang F, Richards JB, Kestenbaum B, van Meurs JB, et al. Common genetic determinants of vitamin D insufficiency: a genome-wide association study. *Lancet.* 2010 Jul 17;376(9736):180–8.

Wang TT, Nestel FP, Bourdeau V, Nagai Y, Wang Q, Liao J, Tavera-Mendoza L, et al. Cutting edge: 1,25-dihydroxyvitamin D_3 is a direct inducer of antimicrobial peptide gene expression. *J Immunol.* 2004 Sep 1;173(5):2909–12.

Watkins BA, Li Y, Allen KG, Hoffmann WE, Seifert MF. Dietary ratio of (n-6)/(n-3) polyunsaturated fatty acids alters the fatty acid composition of bone compartments and biomarkers of bone formation in rats. *J Nutr.* 2000 Sep;130(9):2274–84.

Watkins BA, Li Y, Lippman HE, Seifert MF. Omega-3 polyunsaturated fatty acids and skeletal health. *Exp Biol Med (Maywood).* 2001 Jun;226(6): 485–97.

Wehr E, Pieber TR, Obermayer-Pietsch B. Effect of vitamin D3 treatment on glucose metabolism and menstrual frequency in PCOS women—a pilot study. *J Endocrinol Invest.* 2011 Nov;34(10):757–63.

Weiler H, Fitzpatrick-Wong S, Veitch R, Kovacs H, Schellenberg J, McCloy U, Yuen CK. Vitamin D deficiency and whole-body and femur bone mass relative to weight in healthy newborns. *CMAJ.* 2005 Mar 15;172(6):757–61.

Weisberg P, Scanlon KS, Li R, Cogswell ME. Nutritional rickets among children in the United States: review of cases reported between 1986 and 2003. *Am J Clin Nutr.* 2004 Dec;80(6 Suppl):1697S–1705S.

Welsh J. Vitamin D and breast cancer: insights from animal models. *Am J Clin Nutr.* 2004 Dec;80(6 Suppl):1721S–1724S.

Welsh J, Wietzke JA, Zinser GM, Byrne B, Smith K, Narvaez CJ. Vitamin D_3 receptor as a target for breast cancer prevention. *J Nutr.* 2003 Jul;133(7 Suppl):2425S–2433S.

Wharton B, Bishop N. Rickets. *Lancet.* 2003 Oct 25;362(9393):1389–400.

Wiederkehr M, Krapf R. Metabolic and endocrine effects of metabolic acidosis in humans. *Swiss Med Wkly.* 2001 Mar 10;131(9–10):127–32.

Wilkins CH, Sheline YI, Roe CM, Birge SJ, Morris JC. Vitamin D deficiency is associated with low mood and worse cognitive performance in older adults. *Am J Geriatr Psychiatry.* 2006 Dec;14(12):1032–40.

Wingerchuk DM, Lesaux J, Rice GP, Kremenchutzky M, Ebers GC. A pilot study of oral calcitriol (1,25-dihydroxyvitamin D_3) for relapsing-remitting multiple sclerosis. *J Neurol Neurosurg Psychiatry.* 2005 Sep;76(9):1294–6.

Witham MD, Nadir MA, Struthers AD. Effect of vitamin D on blood pressure: a systematic review and meta-analysis. *J Hypertens.* 2009;27:1948–54.

Wortsman J, Matsuoka LY, Chen TC, Lu Z, Holick MF. Decreased bioavailability of vitamin D in obesity. *Am J Clin Nutr.* 2000 Sep;72(3):690–3.

Wu J, Garami M, Cheng T, Gardner DG. 1,25(oh)2 vitamin D3, and retinoic acid antagonize endothelin-stimulated hypertrophy of neonatal rat cardiac myocytes. *J Clin Invest.* 1996;97:1577–88.

Xiang W, Kong J, Chen S, Cao LP, Qiao G, Zheng W, Liu W, Li X, Gardner DG, Li YC. Cardiac hypertrophy in vitamin D receptor knockout mice: role of the systemic and cardiac renin-angiotensin systems. *Am J Physiol Endocrinol Metab.* 2005 Jan;288(1):E125–32. Epub 2004 Sep 14.

Yan SF, Yan SD, Schmidt AM. Tempering the wrath of RAGE: an emerging therapeutic strategy against diabetic complications, neurodegeneration, and inflammation. *Ann Med.* 2009;41(6):408–22.

Yang CY, Chiu HF, Cheng MF, Hsu TY, Cheng MF, Wu TN. Calcium and magnesium in drinking water and the risk of death from breast cancer. *J Toxicol Environ Health A.* 2000 Jun;60(4):231–41.

Yang CY, Chiu HF, Tsai SS, Cheng MF, Lin MC, Sung FC. Calcium and magnesium in drinking water and risk of death from prostate cancer. *J Toxicol Environ Health A.* 2000 May 12;60(1):17–26.

Yang CY, Chiu HF, Tsai SS, Wu TN, Chang CC. Magnesium and calcium in drinking water and the risk of death from esophageal cancer. *Magnes Res.* 2002 Dec;15(3–4):215–22.

Yao S, Sucheston LE, Millen AE, Johnson CS, Trump DL, Nesline MK, Davis W, Hong CC, McCann SE, Hwang H, Kulkarni S, Edge SB, O'Connor TL, Ambrosone CB. Pretreatment serum concentrations of 25-hydroxyvitamin D and breast cancer prognostic characteristics: a case-control and a case-series study. *PLoS One.* 2011 Feb 28;6(2):e17251.

Yin L, Grandi N, Raum E, Haug U, Arndt V, Brenner H. Meta-analysis: Serum vitamin D and breast cancer risk. *European Journal of Cancer.* 2010;46:2196–205.

Young KA, Engelman CD, Langefeld CD, Hairston KG, Haffner SM, Bryer-Ash M, Norris JM. Association of plasma vitamin D levels with adiposity in Hispanic and African Americans. *J Clin Endocrinol Metab.* 2009; Sep;94(9):3306–13.

Young KA, Snell-Bergeon JK, Naik RG, Hokanson JE, Tarullo D, Gottlieb PA, Garg SK, Rewers M. Vitamin D deficiency and coronary artery calcification in subjects with type 1 diabetes. *Diabetes Care.* 2011 Feb;34(2):454–8.

Yu S, Cantorna MT. Epigenetic reduction in invariant NKT cells following in utero vitamin D deficiency in mice. *J Immunol.* 2011 Feb 1;186(3):1384–90.

Yuan W, Pan W, Kong J, Zheng W, Szeto FL, Wong KE, Cohen R, Klopot A, Zhang Z, Li YC. 1,25-dihydroxyvitamin D3 suppresses renin gene transcription by blocking the activity of the cyclic amp response element in the renin gene promoter. *J Biol Chem.* 2007;282:29821–30.

Zhang SM, Hunter DJ, Rosner BA, Giovannucci EL, Colditz GA, Speizer FE, Willett WC. Intakes of fruits, vegetables, and related nutrients and the risk of non-Hodgkin's lymphoma among women. *Cancer Epidemiol Biomarkers Prev.* 2000 May;9(5):477–85.

Zhou C, Lu F, Cao K, Xu D, Goltzman D, Miao D. Calcium-independent and 1,25(OH)2D3-dependent regulation of the renin-angiotensin system in 1alpha-hydroxylase knockout mice. *Kidney Int.* 2008;74:170–9.

Zhou W, Suk R, Liu G, Park S, Neuberg DS, Wain JC, Lynch TJ, Giovannucci E, Christiani DC. Vitamin D is associated with improved survival in early-stage non-small cell lung cancer patients. *Cancer Epidemiol Biomarkers Prev.* 2005 Oct;14(10):2303–9.

Zittermann A. Serum 25-hydroxyvitamin D response to oral vitamin D intake in children. *Am J Clin Nutr.* 2003 Sep;78(3):496–7.

———. Vitamin D in preventive medicine: are we ignoring the evidence? *Br J Nutr.* 2003 May;89(5):552–72.

Zittermann A, Dembinski J, Stehle P. Low vitamin D status is associated with low cord blood levels of the immunosuppressive cytokine interleukin-10. *Pediatr Allergy Immunol.* 2004 Jun;15(3):242–6.

Zittermann A, Frisch S, Berthold HK, Gotting C, Kuhn J, Kleesiek K, Stehle P, Koertke H, Koerfer R. Vitamin D supplementation enhances the beneficial effects of weight loss on cardiovascular disease risk markers. *Am J Clin Nutr.* 2009;89:1321–7.

Zittermann A, Schleithoff SS, Koerfer R. Putting cardiovascular disease and vitamin D insufficiency into perspective. *Br J Nutr.* 2005 Oct;94(4):483–92.

Zwart SR, Hargens AR, Smith SM. The ratio of animal protein intake to potassium intake is a predictor of bone resorption in space flight analogues and in ambulatory subjects. *Am J Clin Nutr.* 2004 Oct;80(4):1058–65.

Recommended Reading

Bailey, Covert. *The New Fit or Fat*. Boston: Houghton Mifflin, 1991.

Cordain, Loren, Ph.D. *The Paleo Diet: Lose Weight and Get Healthy by Eating the Food You Were Designed to Eat*. Hoboken, N.J.: John Wiley & Sons, 2010.

Feldman D., J.W. Pike, and F. H. Glorieux, eds. *Vitamin D*, 2nd ed. Burlington, Mass.: Elsevier, 2004.

Holick, Michael, Ph.D., M.D. *The UV Advantage: The Medical Breakthrough That Shows How to Harvest the Power of the Sun for Your Health*. ibooks, 2004.

Index